KUNDALINI AWAKENING

THE COMPLETE KUNDALINI AWAKENING GUIDE TO ACHIEVE A HIGHER MINDFULNESS, HEAL YOUR BODY AND GAIN ENLIGHTENMENT WITH SPIRITUAL TRANSCENDENCE USING MEDITATION. INCREASE PSYCHIC INTUITION AND MIND POWER

Mindfulness Experience

DISCLAIMER

Copyright © Material 2020 all rights reserved.

No part of this publication may be reproduced. Stored in a retrieval system or transmitted in any form or by any means, electronic. Mechanicals. Photocopying, recording, scanning, or otherwise, without express written permission of the publisher. This information does not substitute for professional medical advice: emergency treatment or formal first-aid training. Don't use this information to diagnose or develop a treatment plan for a health problem or disease without consulting a qualified health care provider. You are in a life-threatening or emergency medical situation, seek medical assistance immediately. The author and publisher of this book and the accompanying materials have used their best efforts in preparing this book. The author and publisher make no representation or warranties with respect to the accuracy, applicability, fitness, or completeness of the contents of this book. The intent of the author is only to offer information of a general nature and for educational purposes to help you in your quest for emotional and spiritual well-being. In the event you use any of the information in this book for yourself, which is your constitutional right, the author and the publisher assume no responsibility for your actions.

TABLE OF CONTENTS
KUNDALINI AWAKENING

INTRODUCTION 6

CHAPTER 1 THE BASICS AND UNDERSTANDING OF KUNDALINI AWAKENING 8

How Kundalini Can Help..................................... 10

The Power and Benefits of Kundalini...................... 17

CHAPTER 2 WHAT KUNDALINI AWAKENING IS AND WHAT THE BEST AND THE EASIEST WAY TO ACHIEVE IT IS 22

Prepping Our Energetic Bodies 25

Meditation 28

Yoga.. 31

.... 31

Working with Chakras 32

Visualization 33

Practice Space 34

CHAPTER 3 WHAT PRANA IS AND HOW IT WORKS 38

How to control prana 39

Here is a simple exercise to help you learn to control prana:... 40

Understanding the nature of prana 42

The Energy of Prana....................................... 43

Controlling Prana 44

The Nature 46

CHAPTER 4 THE AKASHA.................................48

Accessing the Akashic Records 52

CHAPTER 5 AURAS AND HOW TO SEE THEM 58

How to See Auras 64

CHAPTER 6 GAIN ENLIGHTENMENT WITH SPIRITUAL TRANSCENDENCE USING MEDITATION 68

Mind 70
Body 70
Spirit 71
On achieving enlightenment 72

CHAPTER 7 HOW TO MOVE A MANIPULATE ENERGY 76

Blocked Energy 78
Sensing Energy 79
Programming 80
Energy Manipulation and Chakras 80
Absorbing Energy 80

CHAPTER 8 CHAKRA HEALING 82

Heal your chakras through meditation 85

CHAPTER 9 SECRET MEDITATION TECHNIQUES WITH AWAKENING KUNDALINI 88

.... 88
Mantra Meditation 88
Affirmation meditation 90
Positive energy recharge 91
.... 92
Waterfall cleansing meditation 92
Whole body breathing meditation 93
Cold water cleanse 94
Blessing meditation 95
Healing light 95

WHOLE BODY HEALING 96

CHAPTER 10 HOW TO MASTERY KUNDALINI 100

TIPS FOR YOUR AWAKENING PROCESS 108
WAYS THROUGH WHICH AWAKENING OR UNRAVELING CAN HELP YOU. 116
SIGNS AND SYMPTOMS OF AWAKENED KUNDALINI ENERGY? 118

CHAPTER 11 IMPROVE HEALTH, QUALITY OF LIFE, AND YOUR EMOTIONS AND ENJOY WITH THE BENEFITS 120

ADJUSTING YOUR DIET FOR KUNDALINI AWAKENING 121
LISTENING TO YOUR BODY 122
AYURVEDA DIET AND KUNDALINI 123
HEALTH WITHIN FOOD 124

CHAPTER 12 ELEVATE A HIGHER STATE OF CONSCIOUSNESS WITH KUNDALINI 130

TYPES OF PSYCHIC AWARENESS — THE CLAIRS AND MORE 132
DEVELOPING YOUR PSYCHIC CAPABILITIES 138

CHAPTER 13 INCREASE PSYCHIC INTUITION AND MIND POWER 142

HOW TO DEVELOP YOUR INTUITION 143
HOW TO DEVELOP YOUR PSYCHIC ABILITIES 144
USE YOUR MIND'S POWER TO HEAL FROM WITHIN 146

CONCLUSION 152

ENERGY HEALING

Introduction

There is a buzz about Kundalini practices everywhere from spiritual circles to meditation/yoga classes. People are intrigued by what it is and how it can be used to create spiritual enlightenment, attain inner-peace, and increase physiological healing. This book will help you master various Kundalini awakening meditation techniques to facilitate your physical, mental, and spiritual well-being.

Kundalini awakening is just the beginning of awareness on so many levels: awareness of your own power, joy, psychic abilities, spiritual expansiveness, infinite potential and enlightenment with the source of all divine energy; the collective consciousness and awareness of all people and all beings and our collective ability to achieve transcendence; and overall high frequency vibration of light, love, and enlightenment.

The importance of our universe and the effect that we have on it will also be discussed to help improve our general outlook in our daily lives. The influence of karma and what goes around, comes around will be considered further to help reprogram our minds to a more positive outlook.

ENERGY HEALING

Chapter 1 The basics and understanding of kundalini Awakening

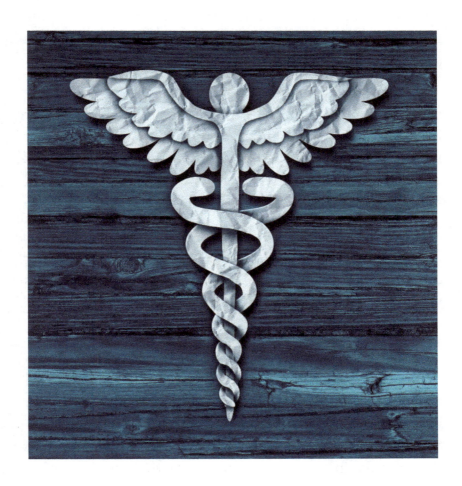

ENERGY HEALING

Some of us may be wondering: "What is Kundalini and how can it help us achieve inner peace?" Kundalini refers to the spiritual energy located within the spine. This energy takes the form of a female snake that is set coiled three times around the base of the spine. An utterly coiled form is how Kundalini first starts off for everyone. A Kundalini awakening is when this "snake" is slowly awoken and guided to slither up the channels of the spine until it finally reaches the twelfth chakra, activating each spiritual channel in the process.

This form of spiritual awakening is said to be one of the most life-changing. People often report living much lighter lives with balanced emotions and mind. It is possible that we have already achieved a Kundalini awakening without even realizing it, as these awakenings can happen from almost anything ranging from simple breathing exercises to a near-death experience.

As is the same with every practice, Kundalini awakening can take time. Yoga is one of the most common practices used in the awakening of Kundalini because it focuses mainly on opening up the channels of the spine.

Our Kundalini is made up of powerful vibrational energies that can be influenced and encouraged to strengthen and grow so that we may reach our higher spiritual awakening. Being able to understand the energies in our universe and the effect they have on all living creatures will help significantly in our understanding of the Divine mother within, our Kundalini.

Some gurus have dedicated their entire lives to the awakening and teaching of our Kundalini and the exercises that activate our spiritual growth. Because of them, we now have hundreds if not thousands of exercises available that will guide the awakening of our Kundalini and the improvement of our mental, physical, and spiritual health.

We may be wondering how on earth these kinds of awakenings could help us in our life or the lives of others. In the next chapter, we will discuss more all of the benefits of Kundalini and go more in depth about all the positive changes it will bring. Hopefully, this book will help provide the right guidance to those of us who want to achieve a higher level of mindfulness and inner peace.

How Kundalini Can Help

The practice of Kundalini awakening is used to help with almost every type of ailment. No matter what the cause, spiritual energy can always help in some way, even if it is bringing back hope to a life that has lost it all.

Through spiritual meditation we allow ourselves to open our mind's eye and see that which was first invisible to us. Meditation gives us the ability to see not only the potential in others but also the spiritual potential that we have within ourselves.

Allow our life energy to guide us through our journey, as Kundalini will not let us down. Once we become entirely in tune and with our Kundalini, life will start to fall into place. We are continually putting energies out into the world and

ENERGY HEALING

attracting things back to us. Not all the time are the things that come back right, but we can learn to control that. What we give is what we get; that is the Kundalini way. Draw things to us using our new awakening and use them to our advantage.

A Kundalini awakening can have some physical effects on the body, including tremors, laughing, crying, and even a surge of energy. As Kundalini travels through the Nadi, it is widespread to have side effects related to the chakra that Kundalini is trying to travel through.

These may come to us as feelings of some emotional trial. For example, the root chakra focuses on security with one's self. We may feel vulnerable or invaluable while we try to break this blockage since it is those very feelings that are creating the block in the first place. Kundalini will guide us through these challenges and help us break the gates that are restricting the flow of the Nadi.

It is essential to understand what exactly a Kundalini awakening entails. Anyone and everyone can reach his or her awakening, but it does take time and practice. Even with this in mind, it is imperative not to get caught up in the same practice after achieving one successful experience. We may try to replicate this practice or specific meditation session to recreate the experience, which will most likely lead to a halt in improvement as our imaginations might start interrupting and replacing our healing.

Twelve chakras radiate through our Nadi. Each one usually has its own specific issue that blocks Kundalini's passage. Again, each experience will be different for each person, since everyone has his or her universal traumas and trials that he or she must face. Once we successfully break these walls, we can achieve a much better state of being, both physical and mental.

The first chakra is our root chakra; it is red and located in the region of the hips. This chakra has an in-body connection with the adrenals and is mainly attributed to our mental patience. Physical harm most commonly causes this blockage. These traumas could have been induced by childhood trauma or even a scare from a horrible car accident. Many forms of PTSD that leave scars in our soul will create the dam thus ceasing energy flow. The Sanskrit name for this chakra is Muladhara. It is also the base where Kundalini will begin to uncoil.

Our second chakra is orange and is located in the abdominal area. This energy is mainly linked to our sexual energies of the ovaries and testicles.

ENERGY HEALING

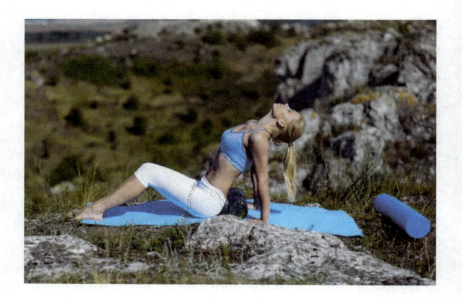

The block on this second level is usually emotional, and the spiritual gain of our awakening here is purity. If we let Kundalini guide us, she will lead us down the path of healing, so that our emotional scars may begin to fade. The Sanskrit name for our second chakra is Svadhishthana.

Third in line is the chakra located in our solar plexus, a bright yellow, known in Sanskrit as Manipura. The physical attributes of this blockage are usually within the pancreas and the main cause of this is our mentality. The gift Kundalini gives us from this awakening will be radiance. This might be a very difficult stage for some to overcome, but with the proper Kundalini Yoga exercises, the blockage can be cleared.

Fourth is our green chakra. This energy is located in the heart and will have physical connections in regard to this area. Relationships cause the issues that usually cause harm to our hearts. This doesn't only mean romance, but family and friend relationships as well. Our fourth chakra acts as our center, a balancing center for our energies. Results of clearing this chakra can bring about a shift in the sense of "me to we."

The fifth chakra in Sanskrit is known as Vishuddha and radiates a deep blue. This chakra resides in the throat and correlates to issues regarding communication. Words left unsaid will poison us from within our physical being. It is essential to keep a healthy state of communication, but this also can take some practice to completely perfect. Chatting a person's ear off for an hour is a lot different than sitting down and making sure we connect and get our statement across. Some of us may be waiting for somebody to apologize or vice versa, but the opportunity is only being delayed either for lack of or a misunderstanding in communication. Physical attributes for the fifth chakra will usually reside within the thyroid for this specific blockage. Once cleared, Kundalini will grant us the gift of unity.

Sixth is our purple chakra, located at the brow. The Sanskrit name for this chakra is Ajna, and the physical attribute for this energy is in the pituitary gland. Our vision is what creates the block for Kundalini's passage on this level. Once we can break through this blinding wall, the most common achievement is command within our lives.

Our seventh awakening resides in the white chakra of the crown; named Sahasrara in Sanskrit. This connection is with our pineal gland and is usually blocked by problems in our spirituality. When we achieve this awakening, the most common result is a higher form of consciousness.

The eighth chakra is a deep black and radiates above the head. This energy ties physical to our thymus gland and represents our power to move forward and begin a flow of change. Reaching an awakening on this level can grant one a type of shamanic awakening, allowing them to project onto different astral planes and travel in their dreams. Blockages in this chakra are usually themed by karma and even the loss of loved ones.

Ninth is our golden chakra, which is located about an arm's length above the head. Physical attributes for this energy are usually tied to the diaphragm. In a way, awakening this level will unlock a form of higher empathy. We should be able to pick up on the genes of other's souls. This ability will also help us achieve harmony by opening our soul and giving back to the earth.

The tenth chakra is brown and is rooted about a foot and a half underneath the ground. This energy is what grounds us and provides a sense of practicality. This chakra is linked to our bones and is linked to giving us a better sense of grounding and our ancestry to the earth. Having the ability to ground oneself is extremely important, especially while trying to meditate or recover from a stressful experience.

The eleventh chakra is a rose hue and surrounds our body, hands, and feet. Kundalini can help us shift supernatural and natural forces after this awakening, and may even give us a sense of leadership and ability. This chakra will link physically to the connective tissue.

Finally, our twelfth and final chakra is surrounding our entire auric field. This chakra has no color at all but is instead a bright energy. This energy connects to thirty-two in-body connections. This blockage will always be unique to each their own. Our twelfth aura represents our own personal, and spiritual path and the gift of this Kundalini awakening will be tailored to each person.

Once we master our Kundalini awakening, we are changing our entire outlook on the world. This shift should help uplift our soul and bring peace of mind and body.

Those of us that suffer from depression, anxiety, or posttraumatic stress disorder may find it a bit more difficult to clear the blockages that stand in Kundalini's way. A lot of these traumas will cause us to "lock" these gates so that our energies become stunted. It will take a lot more practice, but clearing those blocks can and will save our lives. The mind can be a dangerous thing when we do not know how to use it, but Kundalini can help make sure that no harm will come to us if we know how to ask for her help.

The Power and Benefits of Kundalini

Your nervous system response

Practicing Kundalini Yoga strengthens the body's nervous systems. Whenever you experience your body shaking when you do a downward dog pose or a plank pose, this is your nervous system reacting to these poses. The stronger your nerves become, the more you will be able to act in a calm, collected and cool manner when faced with any kind of situation.

Willpower

We all want stronger willpower. With kundalini yoga, you get to empower and awaken your willpower at the center of your solar plexus or the third chakra, located at your navel point. When this happens, one of the things you may experience is a strong heat around this region, and this ultimately leads to better digestion and not just in terms of food but also your memories, good and bad as well as with self-doubt.

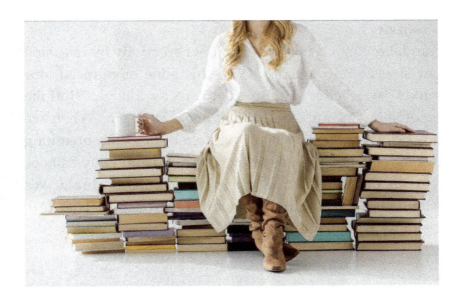

We are much more able to process and digest events that take place, and we are more focused on taking the necessary action to eradicate elements that cause us harm and this could be a person, a thing or even a situation.

Brain Power

Better brain power enables us to focus better. Practicing Kundalini enables us to get rid of the fogginess of our minds. With just a few minutes of rapid breathing, our minds become untangled of the cobweb of thoughts, we develop a crystal-clear mind, we are more alert and focused, and our concentration becomes better.

Our minds are less clouded with thoughts, and we have a better capacity to make sound decisions.

Creativity

Kundalini yoga brings out our inner creativity by releasing our stresses and worries. With this gone or reduced, our minds are better equipped to focus on the infinite possibilities of an issue or solving a problem. When we practice Kundalini yoga, we alternate our breathing through the nostrils-this brings our mind and body balance to both the right and left hemispheres of the brain. We stimulate and use both sides of the brain to act, analyze, feel, visualize and imagine.

Embracing

Kundalini also opens up our fourth chakra, the heart center. Doing the tree post enables us to root our chakra with security, and this makes us feel stronger and steadier like a strong, rooted tree that is planted firmly on Earth. We also become more open and trusting with the higher power, trusting that we will be provided with what we need when the time is right.

We do not feel like our life has ended when we do not get the job we want, we do not feel like there is nothing to live for when the person we love has left us, we do not feel depressed when we fail an exam. Whatever that happens, we go through these situations with an attitude of acceptance.

Compassionate communication

Poses like the Shoulder Stand opens our throat center or the fifth chakra in Kundalini yoga. This makes us more forgiving and compassionate, and it makes us less judgmental. We are always reminded to give gratitude and to address the people we speak to and come into contact. Whenever there is an issue that is bothering you, you find the best way and positive way to express yourself in a way that everyone understands and without confrontation.

Awakened intuition

Whenever we are faced with an issue or a problem, we spend so much time thinking about the pros and cons when in fact, we already have an answer to that problem. Deep inside us, we already know what we want to do, or we often have a gut feeling of what would happen or could happen. Kundalini yoga enables us to exercise the ability to pause and listen to this gut feeling of ours. It helps us quieten our mind so that our thoughts become still and we can hear what our heart yearns for. This will ultimately make us better in dealing and solving problems.

Making wise choices

Practicing yoga brings out the best in you. Any form of yoga you choose to do, you will end up eliminating bad behaviors from your system from removing yourself voluntarily from toxic situations, ending your contact with

ENERGY HEALING

toxic people, stopping negative habits such as drinking, smoking and doing drugs. You will become better and start consuming healthier foods, doing things to protect animals and the environment, serving others in charitable causes and giving back to the community. In other words, you do things consciously to bring out the best in you.

Kundalini also helps bring a strong connection between our soul as well as our purpose here on earth. This is where we start making great strides towards living as enlightened people. So, in practicing Kundalini yoga, practice it for yourself. It will add depth and richness to your life.

Chapter 2 What Kundalini awakening is and what the best and the easiest way to achieve it is

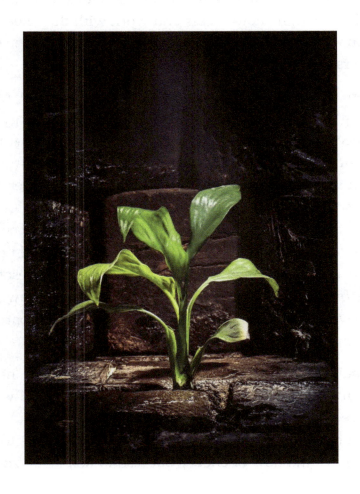

The kundalini energy is as mysterious as it is powerful. When you begin to work with it, you will realize why it is a practice that many people spend their whole lives performing. To work with this energy is to seek the divine, to reveal the true nature of reality and find our innermost potential as humans. These are no small achievements. They require dedication and hard work to accomplish. Overall the kundalini is consciousness manifest inside each human, to access and work with this energy to dance with Shiva and Shakti, unfolding your own personal universe.

When we reference kundalini awakening, we are really talking about the acknowledgment of this energy. In essence to awaken this energy is to work with it intentionally and live with it, rather than separate from it. When we begin to work with this energy, we awaken it, it may still be coiled, but it is no longer dormant. As the serpent uncoils, we find it shakes off its slumber and begins to move through the nadis and chakras. This awakening is only the beginning of a powerful and esoteric transformation. When we awaken kundalini, we awaken ourselves and take the first steps on a holy path to wholeness.

We have seen the relationship between kundalini, nadis, and chakras. As a preliminary practice to kundalini work, we need to familiarize ourselves with the chakras and their attributes. Working with these energy centers helps to not only move the flow of energy but also to help analyze any personal issues we have with our physical self. Meditating on the chakras is a great way to self-examine, almost like a self-psychoanalysis. We can learn about what factors in our physical lives are causing us pain or preventing us from progressing through life. We can learn to live with our subtle energetic body in mind at all times, learning to think with these concepts and make them a core part of our human experience.

This introduction of energetic concepts into our daily lives is the first step to developing a practice that will act to wake the kundalini energy. We need to approach these ideas cautiously, with patience and respect. These practices are transformative in nature, they will change your life, and we want to ensure that our lives change for the better.

We have learned that kundalini is a fragment of the source of the universe. By learning to live with this notion on a day to day basis, we can familiarize ourselves with this energy, letting it become a part of our everyday life and thus rebuilding a relationship that is mostly lost in western society. These small steps to building this relationship are just as important as the practices themselves. We need to acknowledge kundalini's role in our lives, respect that role, and then actively work with it to empower ourselves.

Many spiritual communities hold strict guidelines and rules as to how to practice working with kundalini. This is fool-hearted. There is no one way to start these practices, and not one way that will work for everyone. There are general paths to take when approaching this energy, but overall anyone can define their own path as they start on this journey. The practices are all-inclusive and universal as means to dance with the divine. It is every human's birthright to experience these gifts from the universe.

Prepping Our Energetic Bodies

When we begin to develop a practice to awaken our kundalini energy, we need to consider our routine as it is. Have you ever practiced yoga or meditation? What spiritual world view do you adhere to?

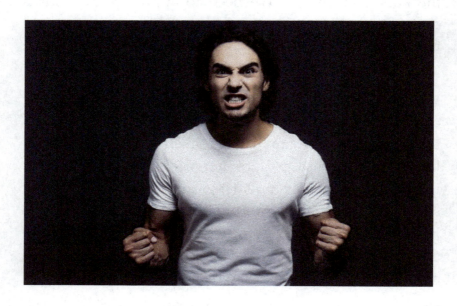

Your weekly routine with work, family, and hobbies will all be affected by your new practice, so we need to find time to organize and practice these arts. We must also talk about the repercussions of prematurely sparking a kundalini awakening. This can do irreversible damage to your brain and body.

Many people try to perform advanced exercises that they are not prepared for, resulting in an energetic upheaval that their minds are not ready for. This premature awakening can come in many forms. Some people who don't even practice these exercises can experience these awakenings. This is common with the use of psychedelic drugs, or other lifestyles that stimulate the kundalini energy. Some people can be leading perfectly healthy lives and awaken their kundalini.

This is troublesome because the individuals do not realize what is happening, and it stresses them out, leading to unneeded doctor's visits or mental disturbance.

It is highly recommended that we start a simple meditation practice to prepare our minds and bodies for the kundalini practices. Working with visualization and chakra energy work are the best starting points with your meditation practice. When we work with these energies, we need to learn how to feel and recognize the effects that are taking place. Familiarizing ourselves with the movement of energies in and around our bodies is key to recognizing that our practices are working. These energies are subtle, so we need to develop our awareness and be mindful of our energetic bodies.

ENERGY HEALING

We can learn to develop this mindfulness by taking time each day to consider our energy. What does our overall energy feel like today? Or what is the energy of the office this day? These simple contemplative exercises will help us learn to live with our energetic bodies rather than separate from them. This may seem very simple, but you will soon learn that noticing the energetic makeup of a room is tough when there's so much going on. Learning to feel this energy is the first step to being able to manipulate and move it.

There are many ways to go about casual energy work on a daily basis. One of the most common ways is to utilize breath. The next time you are stressed or upset, make it a point to feel the tense energy. Really feel its tension and discomfort. Now take a deep breath and see how you feel. Do this breath ten times and see how your energy changes. It will typically be more comfortable and easier to manage. This simple breathing exercise is the starting point of your new path to kundalini awakening. It literally starts with one deep breath.

Let's take time to explore more techniques and methods that can be used to align our minds with the energetic currents all around us. These techniques are not mandatory but are the proven most effective ways to reach our goals with the kundalini energy. Yoga and meditation will be our main focus for the preliminary exercises. These practices are rooted in Indian culture, just like the concepts of kundalini. We can start a simple practice performing these arts to help us ease into the lifestyle that is centered on awakening the kundalini energy.

As we see in the modern West, these practices are often used for physical benefits only, even though there is an invaluable amount of spiritual wealth to be found with these arts. For our intents and purposes in this book, we will focus on these practices to prepare our minds and bodies for our more advanced kundalini work. These practices can be practiced with what we have learned about chakras as well. With this in mind, we will develop a routine practice that we can practice as much as possible to prepare for our awakening. This includes including chakra energy work into our practices.

When we work with kundalini, we can take common practices like meditation and yoga, then include a kundalini-centric mindset to filter the practices through. While practicing meditation and yoga will stimulate your energetic body, we need to approach kundalini directly through these ancient practices to truly awaken the serpent. The following practices are great for beginners to start working with their energetic systems. Let's explore these practices as we begin.

Meditation

The practice of meditation aims to clear the mind of chaotic thoughts and memories. This state of no-thought is the preferred mindset to be in when we are working with our energy.

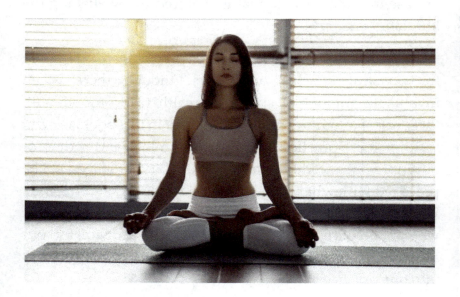

With a clear mind, we can better acknowledge our energy at work. We will not be distracted by the constant onslaught of the chaotic mind.

Meditation has found popularity in the West, but mainly for physical benefits. The calming of the mind and peaceful nature of this practice is beneficial, but we need to focus heavily on our energetic bodies to achieve our desired results of awakening the kundalini energy.

The practice is difficult to define with only one definition. There are so many varying techniques and traditions that a simple definition just won't suffice. The rise in popularity of meditation in the West accompanied yoga and concepts of kundalini in the 1960s. As it found its way to the West, it adopted many different techniques and practices to build a complex and powerful art form that it has become today.

A standard definition of meditation can be any practice whose ultimate goal is to clear the mind of thought and offer a sense of expanded consciousness for the practitioner. These practices can include; breath work, visualization, musical trance, mantra, and a variety of other techniques that promote these ideas. Overall this practice is another universal exercise that adheres to no spiritual or religious affiliation, but rather offers a beneficial experience to anyone who's willing to dedicate some time to the practices. These techniques have been used by humans for thousands of years to access hidden knowledge and balance the chaotic mind.

To achieve the calm state of mind that meditation offers is invaluable, there are no other practices that claim to achieve these outcomes. To achieve this, one-pointed stillness is one of the main goals of meditation. In all major religions and spiritual traditions, this stillness is key to open the body and mind to the unseen natural forces at work all around us and within us. If we are distracted by our own thoughts, we may miss important insights or realizations that are much needed to achieve our desired goals. This is where the concept of the present moment comes into play a well. Many of the thoughts that are so distracting during meditation stem from being stuck in the past or future. By staying in the present moment, we can avoid these distracting thoughts.

Yoga

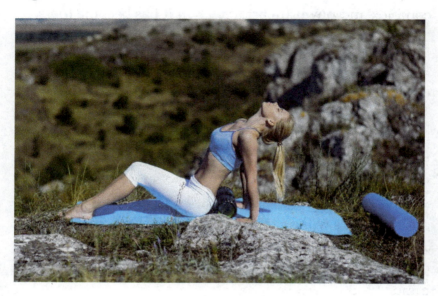

The word yoga is loosely translated as 'union' in English. This is a reference to the union of body and mind. This union is attainable with yogic practice, not unlike the union we seek to induce between Shakti and Shiva with the awakening of the kundalini energy. This yogic union is a great precursor to the union of kundalini. If we can properly experience the union of body and mind, seeing that we are not separate from the mind, then we can understand the principles of kundalini more fluently. Yoga lives hand in hand with meditation. Consider finding the union of body and mind, then sitting to contemplate or simply live in the experience. It is also thought that if your body is limber and flexible that you will be able to sit for longer periods of meditation without experiencing pain or tightened muscles. These two practices, paired together, are crucial as preliminary exercises to awaken kundalini.

Working with Chakras

The disc-like nature of the chakras allows us to feel their energy flowing through us. As a basic practice, we can sit down and try to feel this energy with our hands. Simply sitting with our chakras is the first step to building this relationship with our energetic bodies. From the chakras outward, we can feel our body's energy. Many people in the West know this as an aura, an energetic bubble that surrounds our physical body. This is the energy that gets agitated when you can feel someone else's energy, or when someone gets into your personal space uninvited.

As a preliminary practice to awakening, the kundalini energy is to learn to feel these chakras. You can begin by sitting comfortably and breathing deep. Try and visualize your chakras, their colors, and motions. Notice if you get any distinct feelings as you try to feel these energetic centers. You can even practice deep breathing techniques to help stimulate your chakras:

- Stay seated comfortably.
- Take ten deep breaths and clear your mind.
- On the eleventh breath exhale as much as you can.
- Visualize the root chakra, its color, or yantra.
- Exhale, noting any distinct feelings or movements.
- Repeat this exercise with all the chakras.

You may continue this exercise after the crown chakra, starting over with the root chakra again and working your way upwards. Visualize your aura as you continue this cycle. Are there any distinct changes or movements that take place?

If at first, you do not feel any significant movement do not be discouraged. It may take a few practice sessions for you to attune yourself to these energy centers. As you progress, you will become more mindful of the chakras, learning their movements and recognizing which of your personal chakras need the most attention at first.

Visualization

The practice of visualization is a crucial aspect of any spiritual practice. Visualization techniques go along with the idea that we need to be in control of our thoughts to truly be able to move the energy through our bodies. Visualization techniques aim to busy the mind, but not in the chaotic way that thoughts come and go normally. Being able to visualize certain images or scenarios allows us to be in control of our mind and its need to be constantly working.

Many visualization techniques are performed by imagining the mundane day to day tasks. For instance, visiting a friend or preparing a meal. These techniques work to help us control the images in our minds, thus controlling our thoughts. If we can create and manage intentional scenarios and images, we can better control our thoughts in day to day life as well as during our kundalini practices.

Practice Space

One way to organize our practices on our path to kundalini awakening is by creating a personal space to practice within. This space will act as the home of your practice. You will perform your routine in this space as often as possible. The area dedicated to your practice does not have to be a full room or elaborate chamber. This space can be a quaint corner of your bedroom or other small space that is yours.

Find a space that you not be disturbed in. Maintaining focus is crucial to a successful practice, and we don't want any distractions from pets, roommates, or children. When you have chosen your space, you need to thoroughly clean it and make sure it fits for your practice.

Once it is clean, you can decorate it as you wish. Really make it your own and have décor and items that you can be relaxed around. It is common to have a small table in this space where you can have incense, candles, music, or other items to help with your practice. Be sure your space is comfortable and that you have a nice cushion or pillow to sit upon.

When decorating this area, be sure to use images and items that are kundalini friendly.

Have a tapestry with the chakra's images and colors, or have serpent images and symbols. If you adhere to a certain

ENERGY HEALING

religion, keep your deities and religious items in this space as well. This area will become an altar to your dedicated practice.

The use of a personal space helps us keep our practice consistent. If we do not have a place to practice, we are less likely to adhere to our routine, straying from the path. This space will also act to amplify the effectiveness of your energetic work.

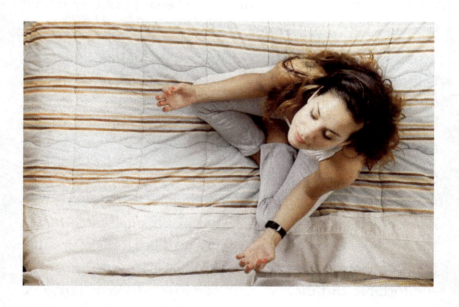

You will begin to notice that even glancing at the space will start to prepare your mind for your routine. This area will become spiritually potent the more you use it. It is as if your mind is aware that you are about to begin your routine and start without your intention!

Be sure to keep this area clean and comfortable. There will be candle wax, incense, and the collection of dust, but be sure to clean it once or twice a month. Without proper cleansing, this space could potentially gather energy and get blocked, as rooms tend to do. With a dedicated practice area ready to go, you will be on your way to having a daily practice in no time.

ENERGY HEALING

Chapter 3 What Prana is and how it works

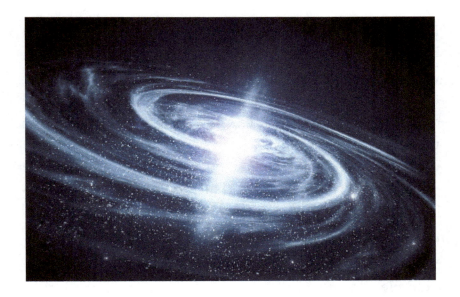

Prana is the all-pervading energy that exists inside you and all around you. It is called by many names and terms, yet they all refer to the same divine energy: prana. Even some people claim so far that since prana is everywhere and that it cannot be destroyed, then perhaps prana is God. There are conflicting schools of thought on this matter, but the majority believes that prana only comes from God, but it is not God. Still, the nature of prana remains the same: It is everywhere; it is infinite; it cannot be destroyed but is transmuted from one state into

ENERGY HEALING

another; and that everything – both visible and invisible – is made of prana. Without prana, then there is no life. From this perspective, it is not hard to say that perhaps prana, indeed, is God. However, this is something that you may have to decide on your own,

How to control prana

This is a secret that you must learn to and understand. You will find this extremely helpful especially when you finally take the actual steps to awaken the Kundalini. When it comes to controlling prana, you should remember that prana follows thought. This means that you can control prana with your mind. But how do you do it? Well, the answer is actually simpler than you might think. It is through visualization. Yes, you just have to imagine it.

However, this is more than doing a simple imaginary act. You should engage as many senses as possible. For example, if you want to draw prana into your hand, then you can visualize prana, like a flowing river, flowing into your hand. Do not just see it in your mind's eye, but also try to feel it, even hear it and smell it. The more senses are involved the better it will be. There are, however, two important senses that you should ensure to focus on — the senses of sight (seeing) and feeling.

Again, remember that energy follows thought. To truly engage this energy, you should use visualization. Through visualization, you can effectively direct prana. There are, of course, other ways to control prana; but as far as working on your Kundalini is involved, then the best way to do it is with the use of visualization while you are engaged in meditation.

Do not think of this as a mere exercise with your imagination. You must also have faith that what you visualize is also real. Keep in mind that prana can take any form, color, and shape; and all it takes is for you to control it with your mind.

There is also what is known as tactile visualization. This is also effective. If you find it hard to visualize and "see" things in your mind's eye, then you may want to learn tactile visualization instead. Tactile visualization is where you rely solely on your feelings. For example, instead of visualizing the sight of a fire in your hand to produce heat, you can just visualize or imagine your hand getting warmer and warmer, even without having to "see" a fire in your hand. However, it should be noted that it is still best to get used to doing visualization using as many senses as possible. Do not worry if you think you cannot do it in your first few attempts. It may take some practice before you can get used to it, but it is definitely doable, and you can do it.

Here is a simple exercise to help you learn to control prana:
Focus on your hand. You can use either your left or right hand. Now, visualize the energy in your body. You can see it in any way you want. The most common way of

ENERGY HEALING

visualizing energy is by seeing it as white light. Now, see and feel this energy flow and accumulate in your hand. Keep charging your hand. You can also direct and accumulate energy/prana in other parts of your body.

Energy is often felt as something warm. Hence, if you accumulate energy in your hand, you may be able to tell if you are able to do it correctly if you feel that your hand gets warmer.

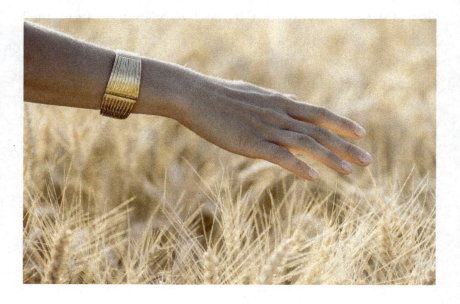

Another sign of energy is when you feel a tingling sensation. This is often felt on the palm of your hand. Take note that energy is inside you and all around you. The energy inside you is referred to as personal energy. There is

41

also what is known as universal energy. This is the unlimited energy that exists all around you.

Understanding the nature of prana

Prana is said to be everywhere. It is inside you and all around you. No life can exist without prana. Prana is also in the breath. Hence, there is a famous practice known as pranayama, which is a practice of controlling one's prana by controlling the breath. Another nature of prana is that it cannot be killed or destroyed. Instead, it can only change or be transmuted from one state into another. It is interesting to note, that conventional science has also proven this teaching, that energy cannot be destroyed; it only changes.

Everything in the universe swims in an ocean of energy. Perhaps this is also how everything is said to be connected. Hence, the web of life.

Prana or energy can also be used for various purposes. It is not just for awakening the Kundalini. Many people use it for healing, such as in reiki and in pranic healing. It can also be used for many other purposes, even for evil. Indeed, prana is everything and everything is composed of prana. Although prana may be seen as one and the same, it should be noted that its quality might vary. When you use prana, only focus on harnessing positive energy.

There are many other ways to direct prana, although the simplest and usual way of doing it is by visualization. Other known ways include dancing, chanting, and certain movements, among others.

Prana is considered important to humans. People with low prana are often more prone to getting sick, while people with lots of prana are more likely to be active and healthy.

Prana or chi has been in existence for centuries; in fact, ancient writings also talked about prana. Mind you, these writings can be traced back to before the time of Christ. However, although prana has been known and used for so long, it is not yet accepted by conventional science. Still, this does not mean that it is not real. Just because science cannot explain something does not mean that it does not exist.

The Energy of Prana

This is even something modern scientists believe to be true. For years, people believed that everything was just a bunch of molecules and atoms.

However, when they took a deeper look at these structures, it was discovered that they were made up of energy. This means that without prana, nothing could live. That is why it is important that you know how to use and understand prana.

When you meditate, your system is charged with prana. Researchers have used Kirlian photography, a kind of photography that lets you see people's energy and aura, to prove this point. That is why meditation is so important. The crazy thing is that the power of personal energy is not new, yet people are just now learning about it.

The prana that lives within you is known as personal prana and the prana that lives in the world is known as universal prana. Both sources can be tapped into and used at any time. Most gurus will teach you that using personal prana is not efficient because it will drain you physically. Therefore, if you need to use quite a bit of energy, it is best to tap into the universal energy.

To help you better understand prana, we are going to look at how to control and use it. This will allow you to feel it.

Controlling Prana

The first thing you need to know before you start to control prana is that it follows thought. One of the most effective ways of controlling prana is to use your mind. How do you use your mind to do this? The secret is visualization. Visualization is often seen as the sense of sight. While this may be true, you can increase your visualization power by engaging all of your other senses. If you are trying to visualize a dog, you do not just see it, but you also feel, hear, and smell it. Feeling is a very important sense to use when you are working with prana. You want to feel the energy as it moves. In fact, you can easily control prana with only the sense of feel. This is known as tactile visualization.

Enough talking about it, let's actually look at how to control prana. This first exercise is only a visualization, but it will help you in getting used to working with prana.

ENERGY HEALING

Start by relaxing your hand and focusing on it. Now, start to feel and see your personal prana flowing within you. Visualize as your prana gathers in your hand. Feel the accumulation of energy.

With practice, you will notice your energy pooling in that hand. Remember, try to use as many senses as you can.

This is going to be a lot easier than it may seem once you actually do it. While doing this practice, you have to stay focused on what you are trying to do. You may find thoughts of "my mind is playing tricks on me," creeping into your head. You have to push these out. That is your doubt talking. Make sure you practice this regularly, and you will eventually be able to control your prana.

Let's take a look at another basic exercise.

Rub your hands together until you can feel the warmth in your palms. Place your hands in front of you like you were holding a baseball. Picture yourself pulling Universal prana into that ball you have between your hands.

Prana is able to take on any form, so you can picture it any way that you want. For beginners, it is best to view it as a white light. Watch it and feel it as it moves and gathers into the space between your hands.

Can you feel it? Really focus your thoughts and mind on it and allow your visualization to take over. Allow yourself to be open to the sensations and relax and allow the universal energy to flow.

45

After you have learned how to use these basic prana exercises, you will start to notice how easy it is to manipulate and use prana. As you get more comfortable with this, you will be able to use prana in many different ways.

The Nature

The nature of prana is that it cannot ever be destroyed, but it can be altered. This is why everything is said to be eternal. Prana isn't limited by time and space. It knows no bounds and is endless. Many people view prana as God. People who can control it have the ability to harness great power. However, in order to successfully do this, you have to have a well-focused mind. This is yet another reason why meditation is so important because it will train you to use the power of your mind more effectively.

Prana is very sensitive. If you lose your focus, the prana will dissipate. In order to control prana, you have to control your mind. Don't stress about this, though, it will come with time.

ENERGY HEALING

Chapter 4 The Akasha

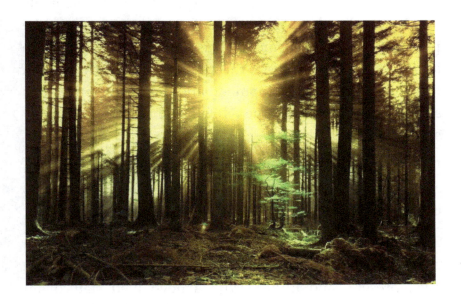

We will talk about the four main elements in the next chapter, but first, we are going to talk about Akasha or the source. It is believed to be the fifth element in which the four other elements originate from. It is the origin of all things. There are some people who view Akasha to be the god principle. While it is not technically an element, meaning you can't physically create it, it does possess all elements. It is most closely associated with the colors black and white. It does not conform to space or time. It is infinite. It is the beginning and the end. It's easy to see why many people associated Akasha with God. They are

ENERGY HEALING

both described in similar manners, so it is perfectly fine to view Akasha as God if it helps.

Since Akasha possesses all of the qualities of the elements and holds all colors, mastering Akasha will give you the power to master the elements. This is by no means as simple as it may sound. To master this power requires a very high level of spiritual development and maturity. Still, it is something that can be done while you continue along your spiritual quest.

Just like the elements, everything in the Universe that can and cannot be seen comes from Akasha. Nothing is able to escape the power of Akasha because it is everywhere.

Some even believe that Akasha holds the records of everything that has happened or will ever happen of the past, present, and future. With a developed clairvoyant ability, a person can tap into the records of the Akasha and share somebody's future. This is the method that many psychics and diviners use.

Akasha lives within the astral plane. This is the reason for the spaceless and timeless ability of the astral plane. It is also important to know that every physical being has an astral counterpart. In fact, everything exists in the astral plane before they are given a physical body. Every plane is the same. They only differ in the types of vibrations that live within them. It is easy to understand that Akasha has the highest vibration of all the elements.

You do not have to master Akasha to benefit from its power. Mastery can end up taking years or your entire life to achieve, so it is important to start using its benefits now. When you start to work with Akasha, you will start to notice improvements in your psychic abilities, your chakras, and your energy overall.

There are some practitioners who do nothing but try to master the power of Akasha since it is the key to all things. However, gaining psychic powers and the like should not be your reasoning behind your spiritual focus. Gaining these powers is just a byproduct of awakening your Kundalini energy. You should focus on gaining spiritual maturity and not be blinded by gaining power.

Akasha is also sometimes referred to as intelligence. Whether or not this intelligence will help you or hinder you will determine your life; whether you become blessed or are someone who gets knocked around by life. Both types of people can easily be seen in life. There are some that seem to get everything they ever wanted and others who work their butt off but get nowhere. It is that person's ability, either unconsciously or consciously, to allow this power to influence their life.

A common practice that can be done to help Akasha work for you is to get up each morning before the sun rises and as the sun comes up, and before it passes at an angle of 30 degrees, look up to the sun and bow down to Akasha, thanking it for keeping you where you need to be. At another point during the day, anytime, look at the sky and

ENERGY HEALING

bow again. Once the sun has set, look up at the sky and bow again. This is not being done to a god or anything. This is being done for the empty space that has held you in place. You will be amazed how your life will change when you do this.

Without Akasha, just like without prana or air, you cannot exist. It is easy to understand that without air you can't live. You need air to breathe. The vast majority of people do not even acknowledge the air around them, yet they are constantly using it. It can't be seen, but we know it's there. That is how Akasha works. We cannot see it or touch it, but it is there and it is necessary for our survival.

In southern India, in the town of Karnataka, there is a temple dedicated to Annapoorneshwari. At the back of the temple, an inscription is written in Hale Kannada that describes how to design an airplane. It talks about how it should be constructed and it talks about how when the machine is flown, it will disrupt the ether. They believed that if the Akasha is disturbed, humans wouldn't be able to live peacefully. When Akasha is disturbed, psychological disturbances will become prevalent. This disruption has happened and we must live with it, but we can still use Akasha and actively work to improve ourselves with its power.

Accessing the Akashic Records

A person can access their own Akashic records without a lot of training or practice because they are their own. This is very different from accessing somebody else's, which takes a lot more practice and spiritual maturity. They can be accessed from anywhere and at any time.

There are some directions that you should make sure you follow. When you do decide to connect with your own records, what is best for you will show itself. You do not have to have advanced psychic abilities to access your own records. All you need to be is alive and have a true heartfelt desire to get started. Lastly, you have to believe in yourself.

Accessing the Akashic records is not something that only a few people are allowed to do, and as long as you have a pure heart, it will not be that difficult. Anybody can do it in many different ways. What plays the biggest part in this is the motivation behind it.

I am going to provide you with a quick practice to access your own records. Accessing your own is easier because you carry yours with you, so to speak.

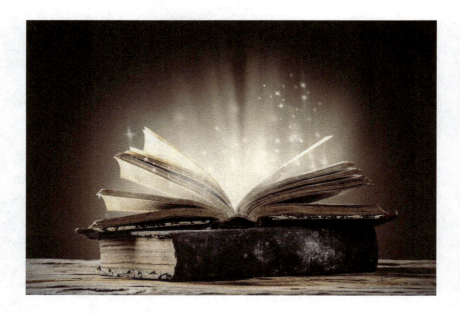

This means you do not have to access the hall of records that live within the astral plane. While it may not be difficult to access your own records, there are a few prerequisites. The first is being able to get into a meditative state. You have to know how to place your current thoughts to the side and be open to the information that you may receive.

Secondly, you must be willing to accept and reveal whatever is in your records. You can receive disturbing information from past lives and the like, so you have to make sure you are in a place where those things can be accepted. If you tend to avoid problems or steer clear of challenges in your daily life, how are you going to face this type of information in your records?

It is also a good idea to have a compassionate understanding of humanity so that your reading is meaningful. For example, you could learn that you were a slave owner in a past life. For most, this will be seen as a horrible thing, but that thought will close your heart and cause the reading to stop. Just because you were a slave owner doesn't mean you were a cruel person. You could have treated them fairly and kindly, but it was the norm for those times and you had very few options available to you.

Having not moved past this past life could be what is affecting your current life. That is why it's important that you go into your readings understanding that past lives happen the way they do because of those times. The more understanding you have of life, the better your readings will be.

It is very important that you have a reason for doing this and not just "let's see what I get" kind of attitude. You could end up receiving a lot of information that may not be influential to your current life. You want to be as clear and direct as possible.

To start, ask something along the lines of, "This (briefly describe your problem) is what I have been trying to work on, and I think there is more to it than what I know presently. If this is true, please send me information on how and when this problem started."

ENERGY HEALING

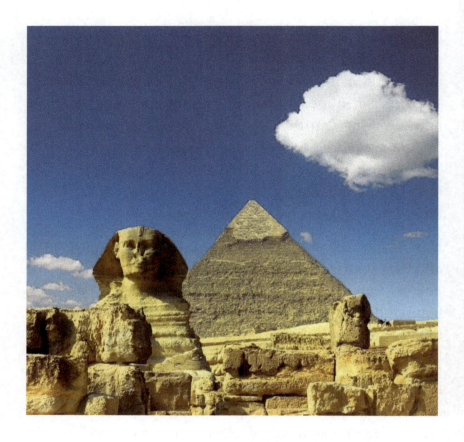

The way you get your answer will depend on your psychic strength. You could receive something from the past history to present, as a video clip or picture on your vision screen. You could hear a clip of music that means something. You could taste, smell, or feel something. Or, you could just realize that you know something. It could also be a combination. Allow this information to come in and then ask a few clarifying questions if you need to. Once you are done, close the session with gratitude. You were given what you need to know in that moment.

You will want to have a journal and write down the things you learn immediately so that you don't forget anything. As far as knowing if it is accurate, you will just know. It will make sense to you. Sometimes people will experience changes, have pains disappear, and some experience a cold before they become better. These don't happen all the time or to everybody.

There may be times when the reading does not resonate with you, but it is still accurate. This is when you have received a reading has revealed an uncomfortable truth. Do not allow yourself to fall into denial. These readings can lead to big changes.

When you first do this, keep your readings brief. There is a lot of information in your records, so you must keep yourself focused. You do not want to end up overwhelmed. This can cause inaccuracy.

I also must caution you this, once you get used to access your own records, you could be tempted to access other peoples'. You should not do this EVER unless you have their explicit consent. Reading another person's records without their consent is like breaking into their house and stealing personal information. No matter how benevolent your reasoning may be, it is still wrong. Now, you can read family members' records without consent to the extent of what is relevant to you.

ENERGY HEALING

The most important thing is to make sure that you treat these records with respect because Akasha knows everything.

Chapter 5 Auras and how to see them

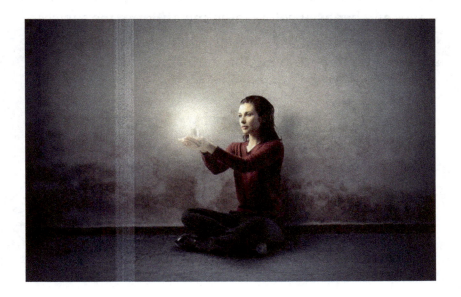

What exactly is an aura? You have surely heard the term before, but it may not be clear what it is exactly. Basically, every single person has one. In fact, all living beings do, but we are going to focus on us, humans. It's the energy field around people that gives you a feel for who they are as a person. Auras can be seen as colorful light emanating from somebody or energy sensed from somebody without touching them that can tell you information about the individual's personality. Reading auras can be tricky and requires practice to master it.

Auras have been recognized worldwide and throughout history as three-dimensional, oval, egg-shaped fields of electromagnetic energy that surround all living and nonliving things. Mystics and other clairvoyants have long described this phenomenon, often describing them as waves and bands of colors radiating out from the subject of observation. Halos depicted in religious iconography are another way of portraying this curiosity.

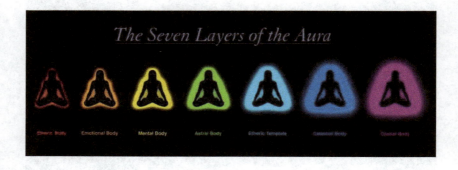

The aura contains emotional, physical, cognitive, and spiritual information about the person, and is essentially a reflection of the person's energetic composition. This includes their current life as well as past ones. The size and colors of the aura continuously fluctuate depending on the current state and health of the being, and can change significantly over time.

People with a lot of charisma have stronger fields, and have an ability to influence people with their power. People who are confident and healthy have more resilient auras, and are better at deflecting energy coming their way.

Those who are unsure of themselves and suffer from emotional and physical problems will have thinner auras, and struggle to defend themselves from external influences.

In spite of these difference, the aura of an ordinary person, even healthy ones, is not very stable, and reflects the ever-changing moods and compulsive thinking common to humans.

It is only with great spiritual work that the aura becomes steady and unwavering — a reflection of the training of the mind. With greater awareness comes an understanding of the value of the aura, and the need to proactively protect oneself against negativity, the same way we protect ourselves against illness and weather conditions.

An aura can expand or shrink according to the type of interaction. In general, expanding auras indicate a more expansive, happier state of wellbeing, while retracting energy is a sign of shrinking back into oneself.

A healthy aura will experience changes, but will have a more durable nature and be able to stay balanced in the midst of environmental difficulties. The aura changes based upon numerous conditions, including health, weather, and other environmental stimuli, interpersonal interactions, thought patterns, emotions, and spiritual practice.

ENERGY HEALING

Another important factor is the movement of the planets. The position of the heavenly bodies affects all in subtle and sometimes not so subtle ways. The aura actually contains the individual's astrological blueprints, and different signs tend to have unique characteristics in their auras that reflect their underlying tendencies.

Most auras are relatively calm with bursts of activity, and are quite small in comparison to their potential. In general, positive auras attract and negative auras repel. An important exception to this rule is when manipulative people use deceit to appear attractive, when underneath they are operating from low motivations.

They are able to wear a kind of energetic mask that fool others into believing them, unless they are attuned to a deeper level of insight. Other situations include feeling overwhelmed by a bright aura because it opens you up beyond your comfort zone, or being threatened by one because it reminds you of your own shortcomings.

Auras are extensions of individual souls, but it is possible for two or more auras to merge momentarily, temporarily, or for longer periods of time in a phenomenon called "auric coupling". Perhaps two friends had an in-depth conversation, or two people were recently physically intimate.

A person's aura can show up as a color or multiple colors surrounding a person's body. To practice seeing someone's aura, you could ask a friend if they could stand in front of a

61

white background. It does not have to be their whole body, just head and shoulders are fine if you don't have a large enough background. This is the best way for a beginner to practice as the neutral background will make any colors that appear around them pop out clearly. Other colors can be distracting and cause bias, so ask them to wear the most neutral clothing possible. Try not to be in an environment you think will distract you or cause you to lose focus.

As well as seeing someone's aura, it is also possible to sense someone's aura energetically. This is slightly easier than seeing the aura, and you've likely sensed someone's aura in the past unwittingly. You can first practice sensing auras with yourself, and your own energetic presence. It is easy, and there are two ways of doing this. The first way is to rub your palms together to stimulate them, and then hold them apart from each other. Slowly begin bringing them closer together, noticing the energy you feel, the changes, the increase in energy as you bring them closer together. The other way is similar. Press your palms together with some strength for 30 seconds to a minute. Then pull them apart, and slowly bring them back into each other, the same as in the first method. In both methods, notice how you could sense the energy of your palms the closer they got, even though they were not touching at all?

Aura reading both visually and energetically is a useful skill for the psychic because it helps you get a sense of the person you are doing a reading for – what they are like as a person and what their current emotional and mental state is. You can pick up on any worries or reservations they may have, as well as what mood they're in coming into the reading.

Having this knowledge can help you tailor the reading to the subject. As a psychic, you will find that no two people, and therefore no two readings, will be the same. You may want to use different techniques, tools, and ways of explaining premonitions to someone based on the insights you have picked up from them.

Your aura is your energy field. It is a reflection of yourself and your current state of being. It can be weighed down and get clogged with negative energies, so here's how to cleanse and refresh it.

Your aura may also be stagnant because you are in a stagnant spot in your life. Do some deep digging and introspection to see if you can get to the bottom of this. Is there some aspect of your life that you do not like? Do you feel unfulfilled? Is it time for a change? No amount of deep breathing is going to answer these questions. If you think they are applicable to how you feel, you are going to have to tackle them, no matter how hard it may be. For your own wellbeing, you need to get to the bottom of what aspect of your life needs an adjustment.

If you remain stuck energetically like this, it will also hinder your psychic abilities, making you feel too lethargic or low in energy to practice with your gift effectively.

Take care of your aura as you would take care of your physical self. Treat your aura's blockages as you would treat an illness or a broken bone.

How to See Auras

Seeing energy is a much more developed and refined sense. Many have caught a glimpse of it at some point, only to dismiss it as their mind playing tricks on them. They may have seen light, color, or a fuzzy field around a person's outline.

When you first begin to practice seeing auras, it usually begins by seeing what looks like mist and waves. Honing in on colors and other details will take a lot of time and practice for most. Those with a natural proclivity most likely developed their skill in previous incarnations.

There are probably more individuals that can see auras than we realize. People often keep such details about themselves secret, in the fear that they will be labeled as "weird" or "unstable", and will be rejected or judged by their peers. Nonetheless, those who have this ability sometimes put it to good use.

ENERGY HEALING

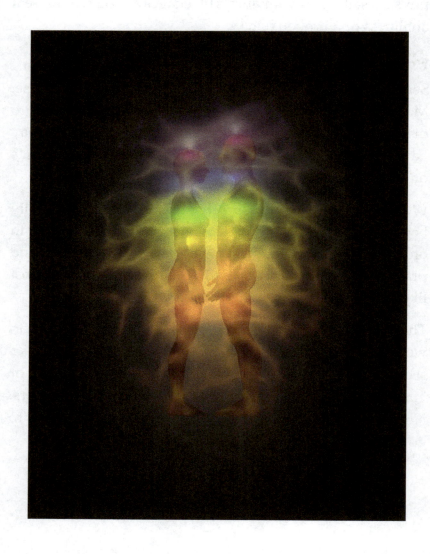

To practice seeing auras, there are certain techniques that can train the eyes to register subtle information.

One such technique involves using the peripheral vision:

- Go into a room with a plant and dim the lights. Ideally the plant will be against a solid, light, neutral wall.

- Look at the plant with your peripheral vision instead of viewing it directly. With repeated practice, a misty outline will appear around the plant.

After this, you can move onto animals and humans.

ENERGY HEALING

Chapter 6 Gain Enlightenment with Spiritual Transcendence Using Meditation

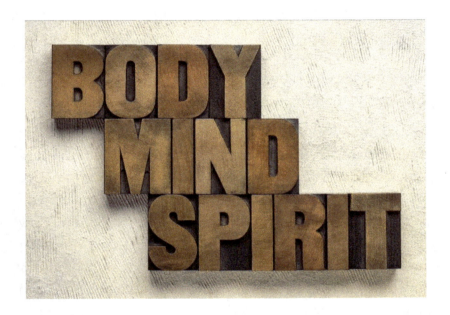

The word Kundalini translates from Sanskrit as "coiled up." This word describes the concept that energy is coiled up at the base of the spine of every person living on earth. It is often depicted as a snake or serpent who lies within the pelvic bowl. As this energy is awakened, the serpent power rises up through the body and all the chakras until it reaches the crown of the head. This coil of energy or snake is the Life-Force, the prana, the divine power that when awakened will lead to an unraveling process, allowing consciousness to shift and become elevated into pure, divine, creation–energy consciousness.

Kundalini yoga is the body practice associated with this energy. The practice of which, along with other meditations, energy, work, and lifestyle choices help the practitioner come into alignment with this divine energy. There are several different yoga practices, each with its own philosophy, mantra and spiritual expression, or goal.

Kundalini Awakening can be very intense and the experience of ascension is different for everyone. It can turn your whole world and life upside-down. You may change your whole lifestyle, or fearlessly start your dream job; you may move to another country to practice your new wholeness and enlightenment in a like-minded community, and you may become a benefactor or a volunteer. Sometimes it can be scary and unpredictable to begin such a journey. It's easy to keep things the way they are, but if you know that you have the power within you to awaken your divine energy, your higher consciousness, and ultimately the source of your primal spark, the energy of creation, why wouldn't you?

There are so many significant benefits to taking this path of transformation for your mind, body, and spirit. Below are some of the advantages of an awakened existence through the process of Kundalini Awakening.

Mind

Overall enhancement of memory and cognitive ability; clear thinking.

Ability to face the uncontrollable and unpredictable ups and downs of life with more peace and tranquility.

Greater mental focus and self-control.

Enhanced senses and perceptions.

Reduction in feelings of anger, shame, guilt, depression, and anxiety.

Self-love and compassion and empathy for others.

Increased or awakened psychic capabilities.

Body

More balanced and healthy function of various body systems including digestion, lymphatic flow, and cardiovascular health.

Stronger and more balanced immune system.

Elimination of bad habits such as smoking, excessive alcohol or drug use, and overeating.

Overall improvement in physical strength.

Increase in energy and vitality.

Can possibly eradicate ongoing or chronic health issues such as irritable bowel syndrome, kidney stones, edema, and skin discoloration due to poor circulation.

Better sleep.

Spirit

Increase in a spiritual connection with self, others, and the Universe.

Higher vibrational frequency in your body's energy to magnetically attract things, situations, and people to you with your thoughts.

Heightened awareness of the flows of energy in all life and matter.

Balanced chakras and inner energies that lead to an overall feeling of alignment and transcendence.

Awakened inner-eye or third eye to promote connection to the divine, experience visions, astral travel, and latent psychic abilities.

Spiritual radiance, bliss, peace, healing, and calm.

These are several of the benefits and of course, there are more. Kundalini awakening is such a gift to the soul, to the individual consciousness and to the realization that we are all connected and have this special opportunity to become more enlightened, evolved, healed, and in tune to our greatest gift of Divine consciousness. The benefits of transformation, enlightenment, and transcendence far outweigh costs. And what is the cost, you may ask. The cost, dear reader, is that you commit yourself to an amazing journey of self-discovery, a path of inner enrichment and an embodiment of feeling one with the Universe.

On achieving enlightenment

Anyone who walks a spiritual path would wonder about achieving enlightenment. In the Christian tradition, this is referred to as heaven. In Buddhism, it is known as Nirvana.

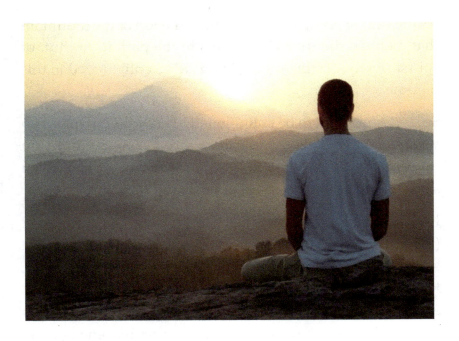

Many other traditions have given it many names, but they all refer to the same thing. You are probably familiar with stories of Buddhists who seek enlightenment. Take, for example, how Siddhartha Gautama Buddha was enlightened while meditating under a tree. There are many

ENERGY HEALING

other stories of how certain people reached the state of Nirvana or enlightenment. You have to understand that there is no single path towards enlightenment. Hence, you cannot say that you need to be a Buddhist or a Hindu to be enlightened. True enlightenment is open for all, even to a person who has no religion. Unfortunately, it is also true that only a few reach this state of enlightenment. However, do not be discouraged.

As the saying goes, it is not reaching the top of the mountain that matters, the true journey lies in the path itself. But, of course, it would still be a big bonus to be enlightened in this lifetime.

So, is it important to be enlightened? This would depend on your personal belief and preferences. For example, in Buddhism, enlightenment is the way to escape from samsara or the endless cycle of birth and rebirth.

In Christianity, you can be thrown to eternal damnation (hell) for eternity. In other traditions, it is believed that the goal of every human being is to achieve enlightenment. However, there are also people who have realized and accepted that they will not achieve enlightenment in this lifetime. Instead, they explore other venues like engaging in psychic powers, so that they can focus on attaining enlightenment in their next life. Hence, with respect to this matter, you should think about it and make your own reflections. It is only you who can answer it. Do you consider attaining enlightenment important in the current life that you have?

People have many different views about this. For some, enlightenment is the main goal on their spiritual journey. Others do not think enlightenment is important. Many believe that they will not even reach enlightenment in their lifetime.

This is not saying they don't need to do good things. You can be good without ever achieving enlightenment. When Buddha achieved enlightenment, he was a very good person before that happened. He was a very spiritual person. Once he achieved enlightenment, his life got more meaningful and richer. It all depends on you as to whether or not enlightenment is important.

Chapter 7 How to move a manipulate energy

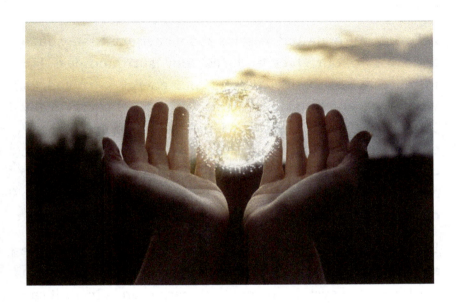

Energy is an animated and palpable life force-one that all of us can understand in the context of our daily life. We usually attribute our low energy days to either bad food, lack of sleep or even the weather. However, the more significant issue is more complicated than it seems. Our energetic systems might be impacted by emotional, physical and even cognitive blocks that we have picked up from far back into our childhood and which we do not even realize.

Energy & Consciousness

The word is often manipulated into defining it in scientific or even in mystical terms and in the process of wanting to define it, we take out the value or deeper understanding of energy.

All every one of us understands about energy is to stay quiet and rest in ourselves and feel our surroundings. For instance, when we feel present, our energy is rooted, or when we feel repulsion or attraction, we feel energetically charged. When we feel like laughing or crying, we feel energy leaving us. Certain situations and yes, people can deplete our energy or even places. On the flip side, we also cling on to people, situations, and places that fuel our source of energy especially when we feel we are not enough.

Energy can neither be created nor destroyed, but it can be altered. We can speed up or slow down energy, and it can exist in closed systems where this energy can help, or it can even exist in an open system where the energy flows. The energy that is uncontained can cause a fragmented or frenetic system. Likewise, the energy that has depleted can also cause a system to collapse.

Energy, despite its power, is a neutral force. It is basically a consciousness that directs its movement. If we see energy like we see consciousness, then we become more direct with our energy moving towards connection and creation as well as evolution. The less conscious you are, the more energy separates from us.

Blocked Energy

Our mind is open and flexible, and our breath is rhythmic and deep and makes us feel spacious in our body. When we are in our Kundalini flow, we enable ourselves to get into a healthy balance that is between contraction and expansion as well as activation and receptivity.

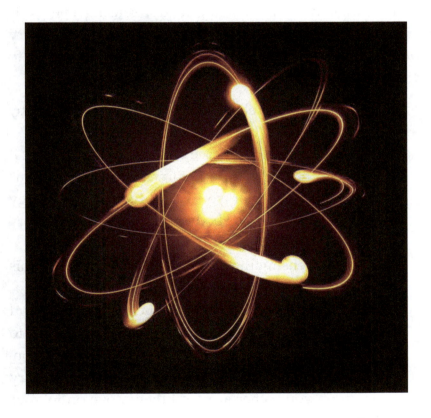

We allow our reasoning, emotions and will to work in partnership with each other and in the process, we create faith in ourselves and often times find ourselves undefended-this is called energy integrity. Energy integrity is usually short-lived, and many people will often describe this energy as stagnant or blocked or even stuck. This is a very narrow-minded thinking all because their breathing, and even their posture is not corrected.

Sensing Energy

Of all things you can first try to do, sensing energy is difficult to accomplish straight away. This is not very common. However, there are techniques that you can do to sense and manipulate energy:

1) Like everything else, close your eyes and start by visualizing your body with all its veins
2) Visualize the veins you see but instead of picturing it red with blood, picture it carrying energy and this can be in any color you relate to. See the energy circling through your body touching each and every nerve.
3) Next, try sensing the vibrations that come while this energy circulates throughout.
4) Focus on a specific body part, such as the arms and tell the energy in your body to course specifically to that area. If you feel or notice any tingling sensation, it is probably successful energy manipulation. Try again on your other arm and then move on to your legs.
5) Once you are done moving the energy around your body, allow the energy to flow back naturally again throughout your body.

Do not be disappointed if you did not get any feeling the first time or even a few times after that. Energy manipulation is not easy, so it takes practice, patience and time.

Programming

The main component of energy manipulation is programming. There are plenty of ways to program, and for different people, different programs work better for them. Programming and energy manipulation work in tandem with each other.

Energy Manipulation and Chakras

Chakras may or may not be useful or even necessary in energy manipulation however the logic here is that energy passes through chakras to it is always important to check your chakra balance and make sure they are not clogged. Energy manipulation may not be successful if you have blocked chakras.

Absorbing Energy

There are plenty of ways to absorb energy. It could be from other people, it can also be from within us. We can also absorb chakras from situations, places, and experiences.

If you want to absorb energy, here is what you can do:

1) Pick a target from which you want to absorb your energy from. It is good to take energy from an inanimate object such as a tree or a flower. This

ENERGY HEALING

source of energy must not affect the energy that you are receiving from.

2) Concentrate on said object and then try to establish a link between yourself and the object. You can make this a little easier by visualizing a wire connecting you and this object together.

3) Visualize the energy that is flowing from the object towards you. Take only what you need and not anymore.

If you are planning on taking energy from a person, you must always ask for their permission first before attempting to take it. Not asking for permission might result in negative consequences as the energy was obtained unknowingly or without consent, which is why it is encouraged to take energy from inanimate objects.

You can also absorb energy from the situation around you. This is called ambient energy and to retrieve this you simply visualize a link to the energy from where you are standing or sitting in the environment.

Releasing energy is often done only when you feel like you have taken too much of it. All you need to do is do the reverse of the steps described above.

Chapter 8 Chakra Healing

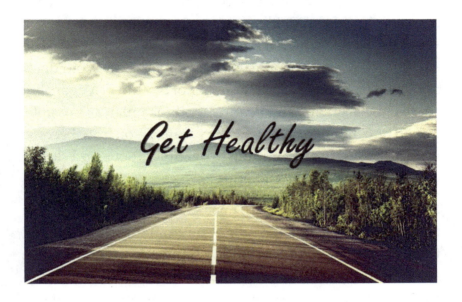

Since you need a healthy chakra system in order to awaken your Kundalini, it is important that you know how to heal them. All of your chakras have a close connection to your physical body. Healthy chakras keep your physical body healthy. One of the easiest ways to keep your chakras healthy is to make sure that you keep your body healthy and fit. This is why regular exercise is important. Exercising is one of the most natural ways to cleanse your chakras.

You do not have to go crazy with your workouts either. Something as simple as walking or jogging is perfect. The most important thing is that you love yourself and your body and shake off all of your negative energy.

Eating healthy is another important part of keeping your chakras healthy. Make sure you consume plenty of vegetables and reduce the number of processed foods you eat. There are some people who say you should avoid dairy and meat products as well. You do not have to be vegan, but try to choose greens and healthy foods as much as possible. If you are not already a healthy eater, you can become healthier by gradually adding in healthier foods and slowly eliminating unhealthy foods.

Making positive lifestyle changes are also important. If you are a smoker, you should stop. You do not have to go cold turkey, just slowly reduce the number of cigarettes you smoke each day until you reach zero. Also, if you are a heavy drinker, try to reduce the number of alcoholic beverages you consume. The more physically healthy your body is, the more energized and cleansed your chakra system will become.

The truth of the matter is that it is hard to be healthy, especially when you are used to following so many unhealthy habits. It does not have to be this way forever. Be happy that you have experienced these habits and learn from them. Start to make small changes and think about doing things that are good for your body. There are some traditions that impose strict rules on their followers. Some go so far as to eliminate all animal products and alcohol from the diet in order to awaken their Kundalini.

The great thing is unless you do follow a tradition that imposes these, all you need to do is follow a healthier lifestyle. It is also important to act in a positive manner. This can be tough when you first start making these changes, but soon they will become second nature. Eventually, you will become lost in how amazing you feel with your new healthy habits.

So, how do you heal chakras easily and naturally? Remember that the chakras are connected to your physical body. By maintaining a healthy body, you also get to empower the chakras. Therefore, to keep your chakras healthy, you should keep your body healthy. The problem comes when you consider how to maintain a healthy physical body. Many people say that you should eat chicken and poultry products to gain protein and other "healthy" nutrients. However, as far as spirituality is concerned, especially if you want to awaken your Kundalini, it is advised that you stay away from eating meat and poultry products. Instead, you should observe a vegan or vegetarian diet. It is also worth noting that there are studies that have proven that eating meat can cause lots of diseases, including diabetes and cancer, among others. If you find it hard to stay away from meat and poultry, then at least try to minimize your consumption of the said products.

Doing regular exercise is also encouraged. In fact, exercising is one of the body's natural ways to remove negative energies from your system. You do not need to engage in a heavy workout. A light workout like walking or jogging would be enough. Simply put, everything that is good for the physical body is also good for your chakras. Indeed, this is another reason for you to be healthy.

Heal your chakras through meditation

The best way to work on your chakras is through meditation. Of course, this does not mean that adopting a healthy lifestyle is no longer important. Remember that when you treat or heal something, you also need to look into the main cause or source of the problem.

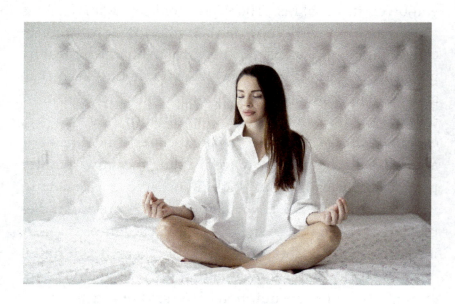

Hence, if you know that it is your lifestyle that is continuously bringing you unhealthy and dirty energies, then you need to make some adjustments.

It is true that all meditation practices help to develop the chakras. In fact, even the simple breathing meditation that we have discussed also helps with cleansing your chakras of negative energies. However, there are certain meditations that work directly to achieve a specific objective. As you go through this book, you will learn different meditation that techniques that not only enhance your overall system and chakras but also specialize in certain parts of your spiritual or energy body. For now, here is an excellent meditation that can help you cleanse and heal your chakras:

Assume a meditative position and relax. Visualize a powerful ray of light descending from heaven and moving down into your crown chakra, charging it with immense power. See and feel your crown chakra being cleansed and recharged. Do not stop until you see and feel that your crown chakra is fully cleansed and is radiating with powerful light. Now, send this divine energy down to the Ajna or third eye chakra. Allow the powerful ray of divine light to cleanse and charge your Ajna chakra.

Once you are satisfied, send the energy to the next chakra, which is the throat chakra. Allow this divine energy to cleanse and supercharge your throat chakra. Next, let the ray of light descend down to your heart chakra. See and feel as your heart chakra shines brilliantly, free from all dirt and negativity. Now, allow the ray for light to descend down to your solar plexus chakra. Allow the light to cleanse and charge this chakra. Send the light further down to your sacral chakra, and feel how the light empowers this chakra. Finally, send the divine light down to your root chakra. Feel yourself being more stable and grounded. Allow this ray of light to fully cleansed and charge your root chakra.

Once you have charged and cleansed all your chakras, see and feel all the seven main chakras radiating powerfully and full of brilliance. Visualize the divine ray of light slowly fade away. Say a short prayer and thank God or the universe for cleansing and healing you. Enjoy this moment of divine bliss and peace.

When you are ready to return to ordinary consciousness, gently move your fingers and toes, and slowly open your eyes.

The meditation technique above is one of the best ways to empower and heal the chakras through meditation. You are free to make adjustments or modifications if you want.

The important thing is to charge and purify your chakras. The said ray of light can be visualized in any way you want. You can see it having the same color as the chakra being cleansed and charged, but you can also just use white light to make the visualization simpler. After all, the color white is the color of Akasha. As such, it possesses all the colors.

Chapter 9 Secret meditation techniques with awakening kundalini

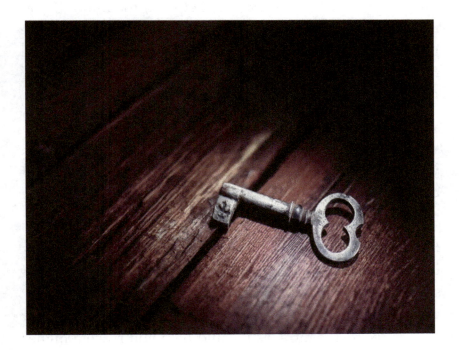

Mantra Meditation

Mantra meditation is probably one of the oldest and commonly used meditation techniques in the world. What is a mantra? A mantra is a sound, word, or syllable that functions as your point of focus in meditation. A good example of a mantra is the mantra OM. The mantra OM has been used by spiritual masters and meditators around the world for centuries. It is said to be the first sound in the universe. Indeed, it has a rich history. It is also the mantra that is commonly used by Buddhists and Hindus.

The purpose of the mantra is to help still the mind. If you allow the untrained mind to be as it is, then you will be bombarded with so many thoughts that it would be hard for you to meditate. When you use a mantra, you limit your mind to a single thought (the mantra).

Think of your mantra as the vehicle that you use in a spiritual pilgrimage. By focusing on and becoming one with your mantra, you will be taken to a deeper state of consciousness. The whole meditation practice itself is the journey, and your mantra is the vehicle.

For this meditation, let us use the mantra OM. It is important to note that when you say the mantra OM, you should give it a resonating sound. You can find many videos on YouTube on how to do this. This is the correct way to recite a mantra, as it could help you reach a higher state of consciousness. Let us now proceed to the meditation proper:

Assume a meditative position. Relax. Gently start to recite your mantra aloud. For this meditation, we will be using the mantra OM. The mantra OM is the first sound ever made in the universe, and many spiritual gurus have made use of this mantra. By using the same mantra, you also get to connect yourself to these spiritual gurus and masters. Place all your focus on the mantra OM, and pay no attention to any other thought or any emotions that may arise during this meditation. Be one with the mantra OM. Nothing in this universe exists but the mantra OM. Continue to recite the mantra. Relax and let go.

When you are ready to return to your physical body, simply bring your attention back to your physical body, gently move your fingers and toes, and open your eyes with a smile.

You can, of course, do this meditation technique for a longer period, but doing it for only five minutes will also be fine. Remember that when thoughts arise in the mind (monkey mind), you should simply ignore them. Do not use a year kind of force.

Affirmation meditation

These days, many people talk about the use of affirmations. For example, when you are feeling afraid, you tell yourself, "I am strong and courageous." The secret to using an affirmation effectively is to recite it when you are in a meditative state. This is because the subconscious mind is more susceptible to suggestions when you are doing meditation.

Assume a meditative position and relax. Breathe in gently, and out. Think of a happy memory and absorb the positive energy of that memory. Now, start to recite your affirmation. Your affirmation is your mantra. Be one with it.

ENERGY HEALING

Do this for as long as you are comfortable or until you have this strong feeling that your desire has completely been communicated to your subconscious. Remember that you are just affirming something, so you do not need to use force. Have faith. Affirm and let go.

It is also suggested that you should avoid using different affirmations. Only use one affirmation at a time. Hence, do not move on to another objective unless the first or previous objective has not yet manifested in the physical realm. Be patient.

Positive energy recharge

Assume a meditative posture and relax. Now, think of a happy event or memory. Re-experience this happy memory in your mind.

If you want, you can also create your own happy event. I want you to fully submerge yourself in this thought and experience it as if it were happening at this very moment. Do you feel the joy and the love in your life?

Now, think about another happy event. Once again, experience this event/memory as much as you can. Use all of our senses. Look around you and pay attention to every person and every being around you. Breathe in the positive energy of this memory.

You can end the exercise here, but you can also move on to another happy memory as many times as you want. Once you are ready to return to your physical body, simply think

MINDFULNESS EXPERIENCE

of your physical body, gently move your fingers, and open your eyes with a smile.

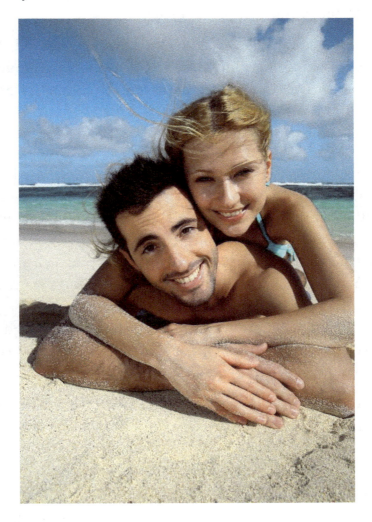

Waterfall cleansing meditation

Assume a meditative posture and relax. Visualize yourself sitting under a waterfall. Feel the cold and clean water as it

ENERGY HEALING

falls on your body. As you do, see and feel that the water not only cleanses your physical body but also cleanses all the dirt on your aura and your soul.

You are getting cleaner and cleaner every second. See yourself shining in white dazzling brilliance. Continue to cleanse yourself in this way until you are shining brightly and fully cleansed.

Whole body breathing meditation

Assume a meditative position and relax completely. Now, as you breathe in, visualize that it is your whole body that breathes in prana. See and feel the vital energy entering through every pore of your body. You are to visualize yourself as a sponge that hungrily sucks in prana all around you. You can visualize the prana in any way you want. For starters, you can imagine the universal energy as white light. Breathe in this powerful universal energy through the whole body and charge yourself with it. Continue to do this until you are fully charged with energy.

There is also what is known as the cleansing breath. It is simply the opposite wherein you breathe out negative energies. If you want, you can combine this with whole body breathing. Breathe in positive energy and then breathe out all negative energies from your system. It is usually advised to limit it to 7 cycles. You can then increase the number of cycles as you get used to it. One cycle is composed of one inhalation followed by an exhalation.

93

Cold water cleanse

Place a glass of cold water in front of you. Now, think about all the things that bother you and give you stress. Whisper or shout them at the cold water. Pass the negativity to the water. Since cold water has a strong magnetizing element, it will receive whatever you send it. Be emotional if you want, the important thing is to let all the negativity out and be passed to the water.

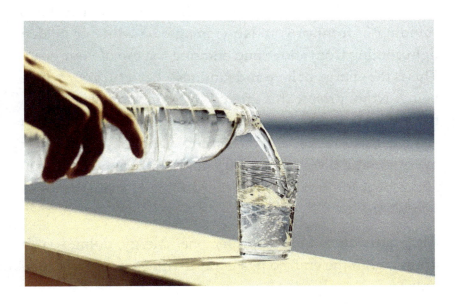

When you are done, you will be feeling much better, as if you have removed a bad load – which you actually did. Now, throw away the water. It should be noted that you should never drink the water that has absorbed your negative energies. Just throw it away or have it go down the drain. It is also not advised to drink using the cup that you used for this exercise, as it has become a home for negativity. However, should you need to use it; you can easily cleanse the cup by washing it with saltwater as you visualize the negative energies being washed away completely.

Blessing meditation

Assume a meditative position and relax. Raise your hands slightly in a blessing position with your palms facing outwards. Visualize the person whom you want to bless standing in front of you. Now, imagine a white or golden light coming from above and entering the top of your head. This is the energy of love and kindness. Let it fill your whole being. Now, project this energy to the person standing in front of you. Bless them with love and kindness. See them receive this energy and becoming happier and happier every second. If you want, you can visualize another person and repeat the process. You can do this as many times as you want.

Although you can use your personal energy, doing so can drain you in the end, so it is good to draw energy from the universe.

Healing light

Assume a meditative position. Now, visualize a white ray of light from the heaven, and send it to the ailing body part. This ray of light is pure healing energy of the universe. It heals anything and everything that it touches.

Allow the energy to accumulate in your chosen area. Feel its power. Continue to charge the said part with the pure energy of healing.

You can also fill your whole body with healing energy. It is important that you believe in the power of what you are doing. Firmly believe that that the ray of light and heal anything. Energy healing like Reiki and Pranic Healing are just one of the schools of healing that make use of prana for healing. Indeed, prana can heal all forms of diseases, but you need to practice your skills for you to be good at it.

Healing is one of the most important applications of prana and psychic abilities. Unfortunately, only a few are truly able to do it properly. If you practice enough, then you can be an effective healer.

Whole body healing

Assume a meditative position and relax. See and feel yourself sitting on the shore. Watch as the waves come and go. The sea before you is full of healing energy. Now, stand up and walk slowly towards the water. Allow the waves stop touch your feet. Do you feel the healing power of water? Continue to step towards the sea and allow the water level to go up your knees, see and feel the healing energy of water enter your feet and your knees, charging you with powerful healing energy. Now, step further into the water and let it wet your body to the waist level. Feel the healing energy of water penetrate your body from the

ENERGY HEALING

waist down. Again, step forward and let the water bathe you completely up to your neck. Feel the cold water and its powerful healing energy bathing you. Spend more time in this position. You are about to soak your whole body; when you do, you will be filled with the pure healing energy of water. Now, take another step forward. Your whole body is now submerged in water. Since you are in the astral plane, you would not have any problem with breathing. Continue to move forward and go deeper and deeper into the sea. You are filled with nothing but healing energy. Feel all the negativity in your system being cleansed and washed away. You are pure and clean. You can stay in this state for as long as you want.

When you are ready to end the meditation, simply take a step back until you reach the shore. Watch the healing waves as they come and go, and thank the water spirits. Think of your physical body and desire yourself to go back to your physical body. Gently move your fingers and toes, and open your eyes with a smile.

The element of water is associated with healing. Allowing this element to fill your body is an effective way to cleanse your system and heal diseases. Of course, this technique has to be practiced for you to be good at it. You must have the firm determination and certainty that the water is a strong healing agent and that it actually heals you when you fill yourself with this element in your meditation.

Take note that these meditation sessions can take longer than 30 minutes. When meditating, time is of learning importance. The important thing is the quality of your meditation. After all, remember that the more that you go deeper into a trance state, the more that time will not exist. It is also worth noting that the key to mastery of meditation is to do it repeatedly and regularly. Do not be discouraged even if you feel nothing the first time you try to meditate. It only means that you need to practice it more. If you persist in these practices, rest assured that you would soon reap the wonderful benefits of meditation.

ENERGY HEALING

Chapter 10 How to mastery Kundalini

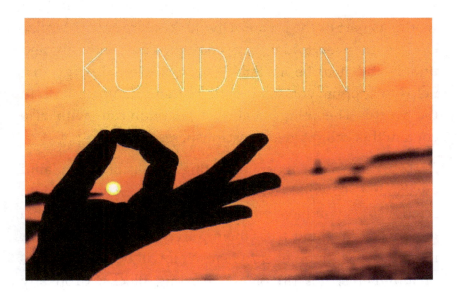

Now that you understand that your Kundalini is a reservoir of spiritual energy and that it gives you aliveness, purpose and passion, let's look at how you can begin to awaken this energy. Kundalini is probably the most sensual energy you could ever imagine.

Once you go through a Kundalini awakening you feel as if you have been healed. You will have the feeling of being able to change anything and everything that is in your life.

ENERGY HEALING

You will have access to an unlimited well of energy, knowledge and the sensation that your soul will not die.

As soon as you have awakened your Kundalini, you will begin to see the spiritual truth behind all things. You will start to see everything, yourself, people you meet and the world, as part of the greater Divine. You are able to realize God is in everything; you communicate with all and understand it to be an intelligent Conscious Energy that helps to support you in everything that you want to do in the world. The things that you communicate with also contain this enlightened consciousness.

Probably one of the most interesting aspects of a Kundalini awakening is what will happen when it works into relationships you have with other people. You will be able to connect, love and trust them purely because the higher intelligence is found everywhere. You will be able to let go of judgments, get rid of any existing blocks, drop any resistance to love and fear of intimacy. Once your mind is consumed with the Kundalini energy, you will feel amazing and powerful because it clears away everything that is blocking you from being your true self with others.

With the awakening you will drop that veil that prevents you from seeing the truth of the world. You will enter a world to your spiritual self, true love, abundance and become one with the Divine that is in everything around you. As the Kundalini awakens, it will move up your spine.

It can feel warm or tingling. These sensations are the energy purifying you and will bring you to the highest conscious state.

You will receive an expanded energy state, blissful love and cosmic thinking. You will be able to comprehend reality and you will know what complete freedom from suffering is like and the possibility for enlightenment. You will constantly feel happy and everything you do, the choices you make, will always be the best.

One of the best aspects of awakening your Kundalini is the healing energy that you will receive. You will soon be able to heal yourself and others that are willing and open. Kundalini power is fierce and it has no limitations. The energy that you will have coursing through you will be contagious to everybody that comes in contact with you. People around you will leave feeling more free, happier and higher. By being yourself, you will naturally enlighten the world around you. This is something that you can really get thrilled about.

An essential part of being able to experience a full awakening is how committed you are to your spiritual path. How devoted are you to seeing and feeling the divine that lives in everything and everyone? How much do you want to let in trust and get rid of doubt? A good way of figuring out how devoted you .are is to see how you feel around people that typically make you suffer. If you are devoted to something, you will practice compassion towards everybody, even the ones that cause you pain. You are able to relax your body which is what Kundalini needs to be able to move. When you are totally devoted to being able to relax in this connection, you will naturally be able to connect with the universe and awaken your Kundalini.

It is a good thing to know that Kundalini lives within you; all you have to do is wake it up. If you were to wake her up without knowing the proper way to do so, you may end up disrupting your typical reality. This can end up being negative or positive; it all depends on how you perceive it. If you have the correct foundation you will have a rather enjoyable experience.

To start your awakening journey, begin by practicing a special Kundalini meditation every day. There are several ways to awaken your Kundalini, but the most popular is to breathe in a golden light all the way up and down your spine as much as you are able to all day. This can be done when you are watching TV, resting, eating, cooking, standing in line, driving, you can do it anytime because you are constantly breathing.

The next step is to accept any issues, energy, people, or thoughts that you are trying to stay away from. These things are there to teach you and a person who has been through an awakening will run to these types of things to explore their meaning and find a deeper compassion that is hiding within. Kundalini will give you limitless amounts of happiness.

The next thing would be to ask yourself what you think is necessary to achieve the emotion or feeling that you most desire to have. What is out there that can help you feel at peace? I would suggest stop running and turn your focus to the connection you have with the divine that already lives inside you. This is living at the base of your spine.

It is important to know that this awakening can be the best thing that has ever happened to you if you are fully devoted, or it can be the worst that that has ever happened because you aren't fully devoted. It depends on how you look at it; is it "for you" or "to you". This type of a paradigm shift will depend on your attachment to your ego.

When you are able to take that step past your ego is the biggest part of opening all the doors in you for Kundalini to flow. To be able to get rid of your ego you have to honor this: you are an infinite soul that can never die. You have to truly believe that you are not just a physical body, instead you have a spiritual immortal. Perspective is an important part of being able to handle Kundalini rushing through you. The more inclusive you are on your perspective of your spiritual being, the easier it will become for you to accept the energy of Kundalini.

There are two more factors that play into being able to awaken your Kundalini. First, how sensually and sexually open you are. Second, how open you are to a spiritual transformation. If you have an open sensual and sexual energy flow with the source, then the pathway is already paved to receive the energy from Kundalini. This does not

ENERGY HEALING

just mean your sex center, but every center that lives up your spine. The bottom three, solar plexus down, is the foundation you need to build. It needs to be relaxed and solid for your Kundalini to rise up through.

When you awaken you Kundalini it can feel like you have tapped into a million watts while your body can only hold 100 watts. This is way you need to prepare yourself to be able to easily accept the million watts with ease. Daily meditation can help you to receive all of this energy. Your body will become opened enough to be able to receive this healing energy from the universe.

This is a lifelong commitment, so start today. Begin by loving how your life is at this moment and start being aware, awake and living in the moment. Treat your body gently and love it as it is. Listen to yourself and give it what it needs. This includes have a good diet, bathing, exercising and treating it like it's sacred. There are likely several mental and emotional blocks within your body that is attached to your ego that causes some limited beliefs. These blocks will interfere with your awakening.

Definitely do not try to force your awakening. If you try to push it through any sexual blocks, you will likely experience pain. This is telling you to stop and work on emotion healing. Pain is the body's way of telling you to slow down, listen, be silent, heal and relax. Be gentle on yourself and continue to do your daily practices. You will end up having better health, energy and sex.

When you open your Kundalini you will find creative energy and you will want to become more conscious, alive and healed. This will make your life full of more joy, love and gratitude than you have ever felt before.

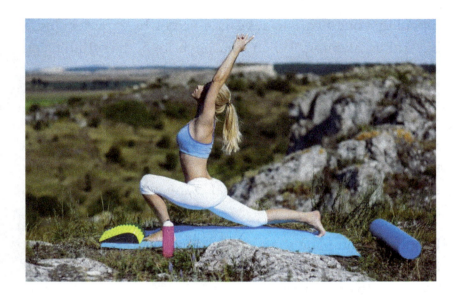

It is important to know that the universe will never give you anything that you are not able to handle, or that you need, on some level. If you have a severely blocked Kundalini and you find that sex is painful, this pain means that you have trauma that is locked within the cells and wounds that are trying to be fixed. BE GENTLE! The golden rule of Kundalini awakening is, be gentle and heal your wounds.

You will find a lot of people say that awakening makes you go crazy, or that there is a ton of energy and that you feel

ENERGY HEALING

out of control, this is just your ego falling away. Kundalini is a fire that will burn away your ego and you will become liberated to follow your spiritual path. This is how you become purified from suffering in the past, present and future. That is what makes Kundalini so amazing.

Opening your heart to love is a secret to experiencing a blissful awakening. When you have love, everything you experience is amazing. Ease yourself into meditation and allow love to guide you.

Your ego is what makes you want instant gratification and results. That is why it's hard to stick with a weight loss regimen because you want it to work overnight. If you allow your ego to rule your awakening, you will only cause a delay in your awakening.

If you are completely and truly devoted to your spiritual focus, then you will have a connection to love and then all you have to do is surrender to it.

Your Kundalini energy wants to be able to travel up your spine and through your head to give you a direct connection to the divine. It's designed this way so you can carve you own spiritual path so you can see where you need to travel. By performing a simple Kundalini meditation, you will automatically feel an energy expansion and will cause tingling sensations in your spine that will give you enjoyable energy waves.

By making the choice to go through an awakening is one of the best gifts that you can give yourself. You will love other people, and you will be able to enjoy life a lot more.

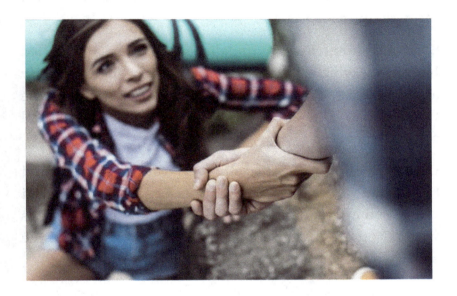

Each sight, touch, smell and taste will have a deeper connection than ever before. It is definitely a higher level of living.

Tips for Your Awakening Process

The awakening process, whether performed through spiritual discipline, or by accident, can cause challenges for you. It's like your body has been amped to 110-220 wiring and as the appliance, you haven't learned how to adapt your body to it. It is very rare for you to go through an awakening before you have completed months and possibly years, of clearing.

This energy's goal is to bring you together with your universal self, non-self, or with the peace that is passed through understanding.

Some scripture refers to Kundalini as a goddess, they called her Shakti, which can awaken and runs through the body all the way through the top of the head to connect with the God Shiva, her lover. This represents universal consciousness.

During this journey your self-identification, illusions and beliefs that relate to your current personality are dissolved away. You may end up feeling like you don't belong in this world. You are instead moving towards a vastness of the entire world.

The clearing is said to be a purification process, or, according to the Hindu, you will release your samskaras and vrittis.

Samskaras refers to the need to work out problems for past lives, or the consequences of things that have happened in your present life. Vrittis refers to the movement of your thoughts and mind. There are several practices that work to overcome and calm the vrittis activity.

You are a spirit that lives in a physical body. The cells of your body are similar to a hologram and they contain memories from everything that has ever happened to you.

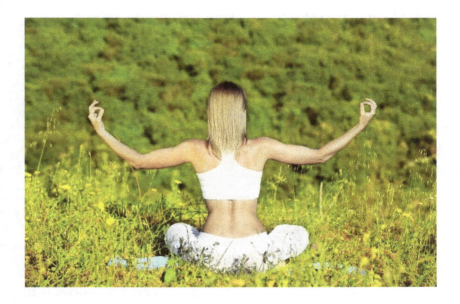

When the energy moves through and transforms the body, the areas with contractions, memory, pain, or energy will react to the change. This is when you will have feelings of rushes, vibrations, heat, jerking, pain and other such phenomena during an awakening. Sometimes these movements are associated with a chakra as it is opened, which is just another way of saying that as a pain is release, new possibilities will emerge.

Each person deals and carries their pain in several different ways, just like you live your life in a way different than me and so there are several different ways that you can respond to the new energy. If you suffer from physical problems that come from an old injury, you may notice that area to be

ENERGY HEALING

extra sensitive. If you consume an unhealthy diet, or your lifestyle puts you in a toxic emotional energy, this can cause you to be more susceptible to difficulties. If you have suffered any kind of abuse, or you have a history of drug use or alcoholism, your body may be hard to awaken because it is trying to clear out all of the past memories. If you have a tendency to fight against things and you like to have full control, you will find that the process is a lot hard because of your resistance.

You may feel the energy as intense and coarse, but it's very rarely painful. Typically fear and trying to stop it, will be the cause of the pain. If you experience a lot of bodily movement, lay down a couple of times during the day and allow the energy to spread throughout you and allow it to remove the blockages that don't belong to you and what needs to be released at that moment in time. This typically takes about 20 minutes and then you will be able to relax. This needs to be done if you work where you are more exposed to negative energy or pain from others like therapeutic or healing work, or if you work where there is a lot of alcohol consumed, or in hospitals. If you continue to have constant physical pain, it may be in your best interest to be medically evaluated.

Find out what it is your body actually wants to eat. A lot of the time you will find that you are in need of a major dietary shift like eating smaller meals, avoid red meat, going on a plant based diet and give up alcohol and drugs. If you struggle with a persistent problem with your energy, start doing detective work to figure out what it is that can be causing your problem.

Pay attention to your belly and heart and not so much in your head. Use practices that help to center you into the present. The best options are devotional practices like heart centered meditation or chanting. These help to open you to experience your deeper self, the eternal self. Start creating more connections with other people. It is also a good idea to start volunteering either for nature or animal organizations; this can help your awakening to be more balanced. You may even find it comforting to call upon an image of an ally like a symbol, saint, teacher, goddess, or god. You can also imagine a golden light surrounding you. There are some that have found success in talking to Kundalini as a Goddess. These are different types of archetypal energies that can help your psyche as it travels through several challenges during your change.

Practice things that help you to be more open. Things like long walks, movement processes, acupressure, dance, Tai Chi, yoga, or anything else that you find yourself drawn to. If you are not sure of what fits you best, start experimenting and find what feels best to you. Your body is what carries you and grounds your spirit. No matter how realized you are, you will be living in your body for many years to come. The more you take care of it, the better options you will have to express your realizations. Somebody who is sick or dying can be a complete and beautiful expression of the divine as much as a healthy person. Poor health does not keep you

ENERGY HEALING

from being able to be enlightened. People that have sat with the dying have said that as earthy attachments let go, more light will shine through. You should not see this as advocacy for asceticism. While you are alive, having a body that is flexible and open can accomplish the exact same thing and without all the distraction and pain. It is also useless to discipline your body by over doing physical activity. You have to find that mid line that brings together the body and the spirit.

Know when you wake up that you do not know what is going to happen and be excited to find out things as they happen. Instead of constantly being in control and worrying about things, just be present in the moment and be ready for whatever may come up with the intention of handling it the best you can. The things that happen during an awakening will be completely unpredictable and will pass, as long as you simply notice them and you do not try to control it or fight it.

You will sometimes experience psychic openings, energetic swings, emotional swings and several other shifts that will be unfamiliar to you. Just observe what happens. Do not think you have to fix these changes. This will eventually pass.

If you ever experienced any serious trauma in your past and you did not go through therapy, it would be extremely useful to release any pain you have associated with these memories that may come up. People that successfully went through good therapy before they started their awakenings

113

did not have as many difficulties. Therapy gives you the skills to express witness and release so that you can move past the problem. The therapist does not have to understand what Kundalini is, as long as they accept that it is part of the process you are going through. What you are more interested in then is to learn how to release emotions related to your past. Make sure that you find a therapist that is compassionate and experienced and views your spirituality as support and motivation to work through your healing.

The process of awakening is your chance to awaken you true nature. Some may be able to wake first and then go through their Kundalini awakening; others have to go through the Kundalini awakening first. This arising happens to help clear things out. The waking up process helps you to realize that the person is looking out of your eyes, living with your senses, hearing what you think and being present in everything, bad or good, is seen and remembered.

Stop being around people and places that create pain in your life. You will probably become more sensitive when you awaken your Kundalini. You will find it harder to handle the energy in large discount stores, nightclubs, or at competitive and tense family gatherings.

ENERGY HEALING

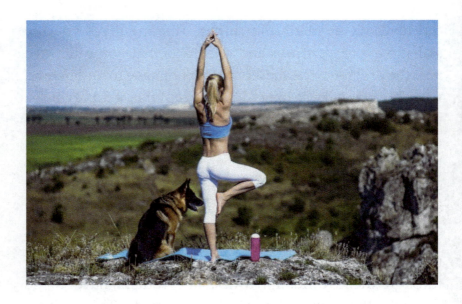

It is perfectly okay to put yourself first and create extra quiet time, more close friendships and possibly a new job, if you find the old one becoming more stressful. You do not ever have to prove anything by making yourself do things you do not want to do. You have to rediscover who you are and what makes you comfortable and what feels natural. Live authentically.

You may realize you have new creative needs, which gives you a wonderful chance to express yourself. Garden, paint, sculpt, dance, write, draw, any of these are perfect ways to nurture yourself and ease your way through the psychic changes. Get yourself an awakened teacher to spend time with. For most, meditation will become a very intrinsic part of your life.

The awakened teacher can help to convey peace to you and allow you to sit in your true nature's silence. Your awakened teacher can have sort of spiritual persuasion or none at all. They do not even have to be interested in Kundalini.

The important thing is that they show compassion and tolerance for everybody that they work with. You will learn the art of being able to sit and be and you will discover the cure for the suffering in your life. With some time you will find the complaints of the body and mental activity will just fall away and you will find a deep understanding to arise. This will give you a sense of invitation, freshness, openness and completion of your greater self's expression. Once you have completed your awakening you will no longer have any doubt that it was the right thing. Where you will go from there, you won't know. You will just surrender to change.

Ways through which awakening or unraveling can help you.

Health benefits – Despite popular perception, awakening Kundalini is not rocket science. It is not child's play either; with practice and effort, awakening your Kundalini is achievable. This energy is known to be powerful when it comes to preventing, treating, and managing several health conditions. Awakened Kundalini energy is known to be effective against indigestion, gastric troubles, and tumors. In some cases, it might also help fight against deadly diseases such as AIDS (in its final stages). This energy may also be utilized against internal ulcers.

Enhanced intuition and psychic abilities — Although Kundalini isn't primarily meant for increasing psychic abilities or intuition, in its awakened form, it blesses the practitioner with enhanced ESP or Extra Sensory Perception, high intuition, and increased psychic powers as wonderful byproducts.

Heightened focus and concentration — From the mental perspective, awakened Kundalini energy can lead to enhanced concentration and focus. The Ajna chakra, which is also referred to as the third eye according to ancient Hindu yogic philosophy, is closely linked with our concentration abilities and focus. When our Kundalini energy awakens, it cleanses, heals, and balances all seven chakras of our body (including the brow or Ajna chakra) to award us with better concentration and focus.

The practitioner becomes a better person — The most significant aspect of awakened Kundalini is that you become more aware, mindful, and conscious. You feel a greater sense of purpose while living. While we may otherwise simply be existing and going about our daily life, awakened Kundalini helps us live (not merely exist) by being more aware of our thoughts, actions, choices, and feelings.

By becoming more present and mindful of people, things, emotions, and situations around us, we invariably become more compassionate human beings. You will learn to perceive things in the right perspective while being able to decipher the truth/facts clearly in all that you experience through your senses. Healed and balanced chakras—Awakened Kundalini has the power to cleanse and balance all seven chakras of the body, which in turn removes psychological and mental blockages, thus making us more compassionate, creative, purposeful, determined, positive, loving, and successful beings.

Signs and Symptoms of Awakened Kundalini Energy?

Beginners often ask how we can determine if our Kundalini energy has truly awakened or not. Here are some experiences and signs that can signify the arising of the Kundalini force. A blissful tingling sensation along our spinal path as the prana (life) force energy manifests its natural chakra healing and balancing act. You will feel a deep sense of balance, peace, healing, and positivity.

Transcendent and inexplicable mystical visions and other profoundly spiritual experiences.

An enlightened and heightened state of consciousness.

Effortless access to one's deep, inner realms of intuition.

Intense mental imagery of deep and profound personal, emotional, and spiritual significance.

An innate feeling of being one with all forms of life.

Inexplicable out-of-body sensations and experiences.

ENERGY HEALING

A more purposeful life with a new sense of meaning.

A complete cathartic release of the multilayered psychological baggage of repressed feelings, thoughts, and emotions.

Chapter 11 Improve health, quality of life, and your emotions and enjoy with the benefits

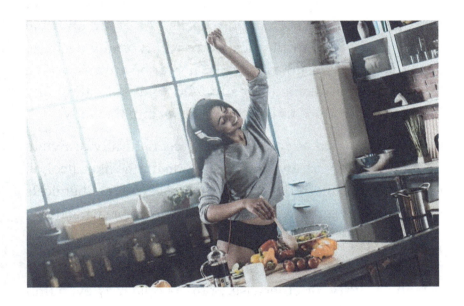

Believe it or not, your diet has a major impact on Kundalini energy. What you fuel your body with is a form of energy in and of itself. Not only does it provide you with physical energy, but it also works together with your aura and other non-physical energy. It truly does impact you on many different levels. If you want to have a powerful impact on your Kundalini and support it in the best way possible, be sure to pay attention to your diet and what you are eating.

Adjusting Your Diet for Kundalini Awakening

Many people believe that to promote a healthy spiritual flow that you need to be eating a vegetarian or vegan diet. With Kundalini, this is not believed to be necessary. However, it is important that you learn to adjust your diet to suit your body's changing needs. As your spiritual energy changes, your physical body will typically desire to change what it consumes as well. Those who are awakening or who have awakened already tend to avoid eating any foods that introduce unhealthy energies into the body.

Common things that you will likely feel naturally drawn to avoid when you are awakening include things like: alcohol, recreational drugs, red meat, sugar, and excessive chemicals such as the preservatives they put in convenience meals.

You may begin to find yourself wanting or even craving more water, organic whole foods like vegetables and fruits, fish and poultry, or otherwise. Some people may even find themselves naturally being drawn to releasing meats of all varieties and instead pursue a vegetarian or vegan diet. That is perfectly fine, too. The idea here is to listen to your body and what your body wants, as opposed to trying to eat a diet that has been manufactured for you by someone else.

Only you know what you need. Following these natural requests from your body will have a major impact on your ability to feel your best and allow your Kundalini energy to flow fluidly.

Listening to Your Body

Your body is already well aware of what it needs to survive and thrive. As you are right now, it is likely that your body has been consuming foods that would keep it comfortable amidst a high-stress lifestyle that may have involved many difficult or painful emotions. This is natural, especially in the Western world where emotional self-care is less popular than in other cultures around the world.

Learning to listen to your body takes some time. Additionally, you may find yourself realizing that as you awaken more, your body needs change.

They may even change beyond diet, encouraging you to exercise differently, use different body care products, or even rest at different times. Being able to really tune into what your body needs is a powerful practice that can truly help you so much in your awakening.

As you grow used to communicating with your body, recognizing what it needs and what it no longer wants becomes significantly easier.

You can begin to intuitively recognize anytime something is causing your body to feel sluggish, slow, or otherwise

ENERGY HEALING

"off." You can also begin to recognize anytime your body feels empowered, high energy, and positive.

Naturally, you will want to begin practicing more of what makes you feel good and less of what does not. This is how you can intuitively support your body and begin using diet, exercise, and overall physical wellbeing to promote and support your Kundalini awakening and balancing.

Ayurveda Diet and Kundalini

One form of diet that does seem to regularly find itself incorporated in Kundalini awakening and energy is Ayurveda.

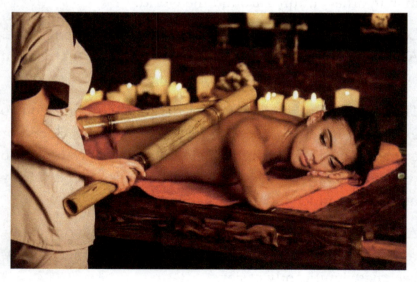

Ayurveda is a traditional Hindu system of medicine that uses diet, herbs, and yogic breathing to promote physical, mental, and spiritual wellbeing.

Seeing a professional Ayurvedic practitioner who can assess your unique body type and provide you with advice on how to balance your energies through diet can be powerful. This practice can help you use your diet as a tool to further awaken your energies and thrive, allowing you to feel your best as often as possible. It is a highly recommended tool to use when you are performing your Kundalini awakening, and even when you are balancing your energies.

Health Within Food

It is essential for us to cleanse our human body for our mind and soul to indeed grow and strengthen. We have discussed the dangers of chemicals and other toxins that find their way into our foods through modern processing and food preservation techniques.

Many of our fruits and vegetables are under the influence of harmful pesticides and genetic modification that can and will cause damage to our physical forms. Switching to sources of food that are more reliable will pay off significantly in the end, giving us the right nutrients we need without the harmful side effects of human intervention during the growing process.

Even the meats that we consume daily, if not gathered from high-quality sources, will significantly affect our physical and spiritual lives. The human body is a living thing that requires careful nurturing and guidance for it to thrive and grow to its full potential. Many individuals have resorted to even growing their own vegetable and fruit gardens to guarantee the quality of their food while entirely excluding the use of harmful chemicals.

Many different grocery outlets provide a wide array of organic and healthy foods for us to choose from, allowing us a reprieve from the processed foods that are commonly sold within the larger chains. There are also usually local farmers and stores in smaller towns that offer high-quality organic foods.

Just about all processed foods can have some adverse effect on the human body; this is why the Paleo Diet is commonly used in the practice of Kundalini Awakening. This diet is dedicated to providing humans with foods that they would naturally eat. These foods make it easier for our bodies to process and digest so that we can take more nutrients from our meals and provide our bodies with the proper energy they need. We must keep the mechanics of our body running smoothly if we are to achieve a sense of inner peace and spiritual growth.

Fast food restaurants provide humans with fatty high-processed foods that do nothing but inflict harm upon our pineal gland and our digestive system. While this form of eating can sometimes be convenient, the long-term effects that they have on our physical bodies are entirely negative. Bright candies and drinks are fused with harmful chemicals and dyes that will inflict harm upon our physical form. These colorful dyes infect our brains with dozens of toxins that hinder our capability to grow mentally and spiritually, sometimes even causing horrible migraines to those of us who are more sensitive to these chemicals.

It is also incredibly taxing on our liver and kidneys to try to process these toxins from our bodies, causing many individuals to live with a higher risk of liver and kidney failure. Using the Kundalini lifestyle so that we exercise the proper diet and yoga regime will come a long way in helping us heal from these hindering effects so that we may live our lives to their full potential.

Water is also crucial in the cleansing of our human forms. Human beings are essentially created of water and therefore ingesting a healthy amount of water each day will help us clear every channel that runs through our bodies. Water flows quite similarly to the way the energy flows through our Nadi. Using water in our meditational exercises to add sound and visual strength to our practices is always a wise decision, but making sure we are frequently ingesting water to rehydrate fully is essential.

Ingesting the proper nutrients that we need through the form of juicing is an excellent way to promote our bodies to heal and rid itself of any toxins. Many different programs available offer a wide variety of helpful fruit and vegetable juice recipes that will help us detox our pineal gland as well. The power of the earth once again stands out substantially in the many useful tools that are provided to us to encourage healing. It is a wise decision to try adding juicing routines to our Kundalini lifestyle so that we can help boost

ENERGY HEALING

the strengths in our bodies that are needed to rid us of toxins and help loosen the blocks in our Nadi.

Juicing diets are a reliable approach to healing and must not be treated as such to avoid overloads in our detoxification. It is entirely possible for individuals to experience a type of "healing crisis" while undergoing strict juicing and exercise regimes. These crises are often brought about by our bodies going into a state of shock from the severe healing it is currently undergoing. Reports of the symptoms of a healing crisis are usually of flu-like tendencies with excess sweating, mainly from the hands and feet. This crisis is all because our bodies are putting their full energy into fighting and detoxifying whatever ailments is that are influencing us.

Our bodies will try to rid itself of all toxins through in any way it can during these crises, and horrible sweat waves are the most common and one of the fastest ways for our bodies to expel these ailments. Healing crises can sometimes lead to excess urination and even vomiting.

The fact of healing crises should never deter those from attempting ways to bring about natural detoxification, as they usually are strictly related to pushing ourselves beyond our limit and trying to speed up the healing process. If we take in too much of the powerful tools that detox and clear our blocks, our bodies will need to react just as fast and just as potently. Thus, if we make sure to monitor our practices and diets so that they gradually introduced into our lives, we can avoid situations that might prove more difficult for us to heal.

Activated charcoal is an excellent supplement that will absorb any toxins that reside within our circulatory system. Taking this supplement in the form of pills or even using the power with water to create a detoxifying paste is usually guaranteed to perform with excellent results. Activated charcoal is a frequent ingredient in many favorite beauty products today, especially common in facemasks and bath soaks. These detoxifying properties will help cleanse our skin as well, providing ease to ailments ranging from acne to bee stings or spider bites.

For those of us who struggle with muscle and joint pain, Kundalini exercises will strengthen our mind and bodies, but sometimes these pangs of discomfort can grow stronger after our practice. The use of Arnica gel combined with peppermint oil is an excellent determent to the aches in our bodies. After our Kundalini yoga exercises, using arnica and peppermint on our usual, or even new, sore muscles and joints will significantly lower their pain level.

ENERGY HEALING

MINDFULNESS EXPERIENCE

Chapter 12 Elevate a higher state of consciousness with kundalini

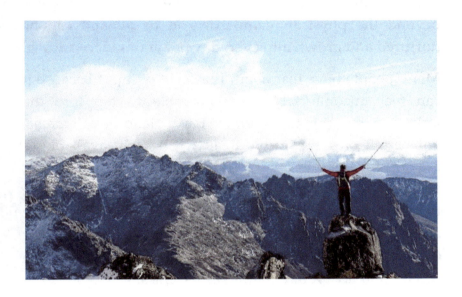

Have you ever had a feeling about something and you just know what others might not feel, or see? Have you ever heard the thoughts of another, but second-guessed that you did? Have you had a dream before that come true days later? Do you ever feel the presence of things that are not of the earthly realm? This is just scratching the surface of some of the things that begin to happen when you awaken your psychic awareness.

As part of Kundalini rising and the process of clearing and releasing blockages and negativity from your subtle body, you shift your perception of reality to the extent that you are able to crack open your latent abilities to receive input from other dimensions. This ability is not reserved for a select few or passed down genetically through generations, although that has been known to happen. This power to feel beyond the physical realm exists in us all and can be nurtured and grown into everyday use and understanding.

Many people have fear about this level of input because it can feel uncomfortable or vulnerable to tap into the unknown, into things that on the Earth plane we call magic, witchcraft, or superstition. Really, it is truly available to anyone to use this ability. When we are locked in our sleeping state (pre-kundalini rising), we cannot fathom the possibilities of such an existence, but as we allow our awakening to progress fully and reach the state of higher consciousness, we can open the brow and crown chakras to receive and accept our abilities as psychics.

These abilities can manifest in a variety of ways and have been reported as some of the side effects of the awakening process.

The next few subchapters will go into greater detail about the different kinds of psychic abilities that can be awakened, as well as techniques for opening and expanding these abilities.

Types of Psychic Awareness — The Clairs and More

Kundalini Awakening is all energy and when you begin clearing all the blocks and wounds, negative vibrations and old programming, you rebalance your true energy and become a clear channel of energetic flow. In the language of psychic capabilities, having clearness relates directly to each of the many forms of psychic understanding. You have to be clear (Clair) to work with these powers.

Once you have opened your Kundalini energy and you begin to experience the impact and effects of clearing your energy field, your latent psychic abilities can start to surface and may manifest in one, some, or all of the following ways:

- Clairsentience - This psychic ability simply means 'clear sense'. It is a knowing, or sudden understanding of emotion, or physical feelings from someone outside of yourself. It can also be a place like a building, a shop, someone's house, and you get a feeling about it and just know that it is comfortable, or unsafe, or has a negative history, or something bad happened there. This is sensing what is not seen but is very present.

- Clairaudience - Audience refers to audio and audio refers to sound. The clear hearing or clairaudience describes the ability to channel energy in the form of hearing tones, music, words, thoughts, and information from spiritual guidance, angels, and even loved ones who have crossed over.

- Claircognizance - Cognizance is the term relating to knowledge and awareness. Clear knowing is similar to clairsentience, except that claircognizance is knowing some form of knowledge without studying it or being told by another. It is knowing of information, while clear sensing has more to do with feelings.

- Clairvoyance - This sense involves the ability to clearly 'see', which often occurs in the form of inner visions through the mind's eye, or the ability to perceive auras of people, objects, animals, etc. This can also relate to clearly seeing the energy of spiritual entities, or spirit guides, but this visioning can also occur, again, in the mind's eye. The images seen in the third eye chakra can appear as clearly as a photograph or a movie.

- Clairscentist - This sense pertains to an ability to clearly smell scents from a spiritual distance. It may mean picking up on smells such as tobacco, lemon zest, or roses, because of their association with people close to you in your life, or who have crossed over and are sending you a message. It could merely be a sense of people you are about to come in contact to or a collection of energies.

- Clairgustant- The sense of taste can be connected to your psychic sense, allowing you to taste something not of your own sense of taste, nothing you ate or drank, but someone else's. This could happen if you are doing an intuitive reading for someone, or you are at a cocktail party and you know what the person you just met had from the hors-d'oeuvre tray.

- Clairtangency - This sense describes a clear touch. For people with this sense, they can pick up an object and know its history, where it was made, whether it was well cared for, who owned it, etc., or they can just get a positive, or negative sense about the object. It also works with touching another person. For example, laying a caring hand on the shoulder of a person you are offering compassion to and feeling all of their emotions, fears, sorrows, and so forth. Another word used to describe this ability is psychometry.

- Clairempathy - This sense allows for the ability to clearly understand emotions. This is sometimes considered a form of telepathic communication, as though you can tap into the brain wave energy of someone's emotional experience. It can relate to animals and places, as well as humans and is a direct understanding of your own emotional state and from there, a sense of another's internal attitude or emotion.

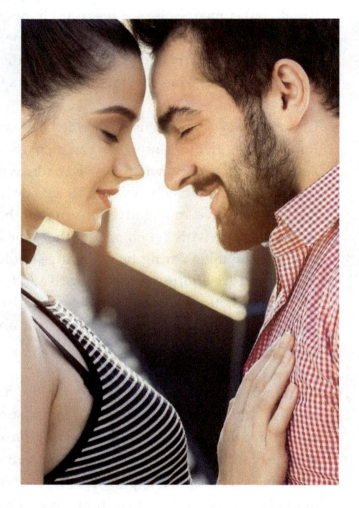

- Telepathy - Telepathy is scientifically proven to exist not only in humans but animals as well. When you are vibrating at a high frequency and your channels are clear, you can connect to another through brain waves which go from Beta (consciousness and reasoning), through Alpha (deep relaxed states), to Theta (light sleep/meditation) and finally on to Delta (deep sleep). Another brain wave measurement, Gamma, is the 'insight' brain wave that allows for eureka moments, and enlightened consciousness.

- In telepathy, you can fall into rhythm with another person's brain wave patterns and communicate thoughts, feelings, ideas, and images. This is easier in an alpha or theta state so that your logical mind (beta) won't reject the concept.

- Projection - The practice, or ability to project one's energetic body (astral/subtle) into other places, realities, or dimensions. It can be just a sense of these places, or experiences, though some have reported what feels akin to an 'out of body' experience (which makes perfect sense if your subtle body leaves your physical body to go on a trip). This travel, or projected experience, can also occur in the third eye and can be associated with clairvoyance, where you visit these inner realms in that chakra.

- Precognition - This is the ability to 'see into the future', essentially. Often, people with this power will have premonitory dreams that manifest in reality later. For the developing precognitive, it is important to study the symbolism of dreams and to not take them literally, but as messages of the higher self or angelic realms in the form of archetypal and symbolic imagery where your brain can understand and process. It can also manifest as an ability to just feel or know that an event, or situation is about to take place. For example, having a feeling that a guest is about to arrive and knock on your door, without any previous knowledge.

As you begin to develop your psychic senses through your awakening, you will discover that there are unlimited possibilities for how they can show up in your life based on your unique personality, characteristics, and background. Do not feel discouraged if this part of your awakening takes longer to know. It is important that if you are interested in working with your latent psychic capabilities that your intentions using these powers are for good and nothing else. Desiring psychic awareness to manipulate others, create disempowered feelings in other souls, or to serve only the self, will create negative energy blocks in your chakras which may prevent your ability to work well with this ability and hinder your awakening journey. The more you know about all of the above capabilities and how to nurture them, the clearer your knowing of enlightenment and oneness with the whole universe.

Developing Your Psychic Capabilities

Finding the appropriate lessons to exercise your psychic awareness can be challenging. There is plenty of misinformation on the world wide web, and sometimes the resources found in books are hard to find. There are, however, the right sources of information and it is up to you to follow the trail of breadcrumbs.

Step 1: Let the Information Come to You

I realize the idea of waiting for the information you need to find you sound a bit wacky, and if you are feeling any impatience to get started, untimely. Often, when we are opening our psychic awareness, it involves working with the energies of the Universe to be a guide to the right source. Has someone ever given you a book out of the blue and said they thought you just needed to have it? Have you been looking for something and it shows up out of nowhere in your email or conversations?

When you are on the awakened path and you are cultivating your psychic awareness, it is important to allow the information to come to you. The Universe knows what you are searching for, and indeed, what you are ready for next on your journey. So just practice openness so you can be aware when these things pop up. Your intuition will confirm you are on the right track. Trust it.

Another way this can manifest is in the way of claircognizance, clairsentience, and clairaudience. Pay

ENERGY HEALING

attention to the message you are receiving from other realms, dreams, and your own intuition and inner knowing. Your psychic abilities will develop in tandem with you looking for ways to practice them.

Step 2: Clair-Anything Means Clear Energy

If you are going to work on nurturing your emerging psychic senses, it is important that you remain energetically clear so that you do not misread or misinterpret messages, or emotions. Throughout this book, there have been several levels of energy clearing methods and techniques, without which Kundalini awakening and enlightenment would not be possible. Energy is key. If your channels are blocked from your own, or other people's negative vibrations, you will have a harder time giving and receiving psychically.

Developing an energy clearing ritual for everyday use can be very beneficial. This could be as simple as using sage, or incense to smudge or cleanse your home and body after several people have been around you and brought their own negative vibrations into your space. This can energetically disrupt your ability to clearly 'see'. Salty baths can be very helpful, as well as spending time alone in nature to recharge and ground your energy.

You can do these things before you engage with any exercises to develop your psychic awareness, or just in general, to keep your vibration elevated for your awakening process. Incorporate some of the yoga postures and breathing exercises to help keep your channels clear too.

Step 3: Trust Your Own Knowing

It seems like magic, to go from being unawakened and in no way psychic, to being enlightened, full of love and light and able to tap into the energies of all existence through clairsentience and other means. When these things start opening up inside of you and manifesting in your reality, since you have never felt it before, it might feel odd, uncomfortable, or scary. Many people can be ostracized by our society and called crazy or schizophrenic because they can hear, or see what no one else can. Imagine if those abilities were nurtured instead of medicated and cut off.

No one will have a Kundalini awakening experience quite like yours. The journey will bring you closer to humanity and the whole Universe, but it will be your soul's road to travel. Self-trust is invaluable along this path. Your quest as an awakened soul is to know and trust your divine truth and honor your creative power.

Opening your psychic sense or sixth sense as it is often called demands your trust. Trust your visions and projections. They are your reality. Trust your sense of something. Trust your connection to otherworldly beings and energies. They are here to help you and offer guidance. Do not ignore it when you hear it, see it, sense it, feel it,

ENERGY HEALING

know it. That is your gift and it is yours to share with the good intention of all.

A word of caution on opening these abilities into your life: check your ego at the gate. This is nothing to brag about. Anyone can do this, especially when they release their Kundalini energy and experience awakening. There is little room for big heads in using your psychic light. You need to have plenty of space in that head to help others in need.

Step 4: Collaborate with the Cosmos
Enlightenment is free. Transcendence is for everyone. It crosses time and space and all realities. There is not a person alive on this Earth who does not share your ability to know this truth. Awakening comes to all those who seek it and answer its call. Connecting to the other realms of life, forces of nature and cosmic beings is an answer to your soul's desire to know all.

Believe you are known by all that is, by the Universe. Ask to know and you shall receive knowledge. Speak to your knowledge, speak to your energy, tap into your light and primal force. It is always talking and when you speak, listen, and then you will hear the answer.

Chapter 13 Increase Psychic Intuition and Mind Power

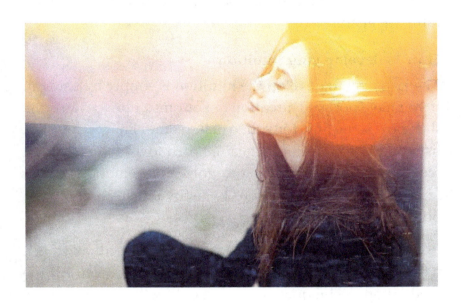

Many people are familiar with what the intuition is, but what exactly is the intuition? Some people say that it is the highest form of intelligence. Intuition is the ability to know something without evidence or analysis. It is about knowing. Sometimes, when the phone rings, you simply know who is calling.

The truth is that the intuition is very common. Unfortunately, today, people do not recognize it. Many people do not take notice of the messages from their intuition and only rely on logic or the use of reasons. Hence, they fail to listen to what the intuition tells them. Once they get used to shutting down their intuition, then they reach the point where they can no longer hear or notice it. The good news is that it is never too late to learn to listen to your intuition again.

How to develop your intuition

The best way to develop the intuition is simply by using it. If you have not paid attention to your intuition for too long, then now is the time for you to make some changes and start listening to your intuition again. Learn to listen to how you feel. A good approach is to recognize your emotion or "gut feeling" and then use reasons to justify it instead of relying on reasons alone.

It is also worth noting that the practice of meditation is a natural and effective way to develop the intuition. All the meditation techniques in this book will develop your intuition. Here is another interesting exercise that can enhance your intuition:

Use your intuition in your daily life. For example, when the phone rings, try to "guess" who is calling. When you are at the supermarket or when driving, visualize the first person whom you will see before you take a turn. There are many other ways to put your intuition into work. The important thing is to make use of it regularly. Do not be discouraged if you commit mistakes. The more times that you use your intuition, the more you will get good at it.

How to Develop Your Psychic Abilities

Enhance your psychic abilities.

We have already discussed notable psychic abilities that you can learn. Now, how do you enhance these abilities? Well, just like with any other skill, you simply have to keep on practicing them. When you say practice, it means actually putting it into real application. The best way to practice is to incorporate your psychic abilities in your everyday life.

So, how do you live with psychic abilities? Simply make them a natural part of who you are as a person. After all, there is no good reason for you to hide them. However, it should be noted that you should not boast about your abilities, and you should not use them for evil purposes. Let us now discuss effective ways on how to enhance your psychic abilities by making them a part of your everyday life:

When you take a bath, do not just clean your physical body, but also make an effort to cleanse all negative energies of your astral body. Visualize that as you clean your physical body, you also clean all negativities and impurities in your soul. See and feel the negative energies being washed away by the water and go in down the drain. Visualize yourself shining brightly.

If you have time to focus on your breath, then you can cleanse and charge yourself at any time. As you inhale, visualize positive energy entering your body. When you exhale, see and feel the negative energies being released from your body.

When someone calls you on the phone, take a moment to define who it is. Close your eyes or just focus, listen to your intuition, and then focus on who it is.

When you are engaged in a conversation, do not just listen to the words that the other person is telling you. You should also connect to them on a deeper level by using your empathic ability. Use whatever technique you may find helpful or necessary.

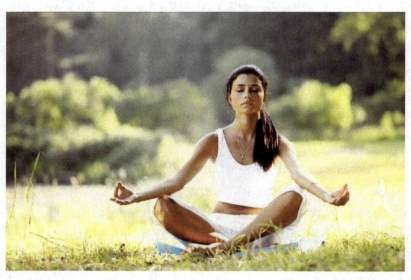

Make sure to make time to meditate regularly (every day). Meditation plays a very important role in your spiritual development, especially in the awakening of the Kundalini.

When you see an interesting object, especially if it is an old object, hold it in your hand, feel it, and allow your intuition to tell you the history of the object. This ability is known as psychometry.

Start using your intuition. This does not mean that you should no longer use logic or reasons, but you should also pay attention to what your intuition tells you.

Improve yourself by working on corresponding chakras.
There are many ways to incorporate your practices in your daily life. The problem is that there are people who simply do not take the efforts to practice their abilities. It is also advised that you give yourself even just an hour from time to time to do nothing but to practice your abilities. You do not have to develop all your psychic abilities all at once. If you want, you can just focus on one or two abilities at a time.

The more that you make good use of your abilities, the more that you can develop them. The key here is repetition. This is why continuous practice is very important. You also have to give it your focus and attention. Always do your best.

Use Your Mind's Power to Heal from Within
Your mind is one of your most powerful assets. However, most people do not know where to begin when it comes to harnessing it. The good news is that harnessing the depths of your mind and their power is not hard. It is all about knowing which strategies are most effective and how to use them.

ENERGY HEALING

You want to start by expanding your awareness. This will make it much easier for both information and energy to start flowing through your mind. You will have a lesser vulnerability to toxic and negative emotions and it will be much easier to process information and take advantage of the energy inside you. Bad habits that you want to break, such as smoking cigarettes or overeating, are much easier to tackle when you are using the full power of your mind and have a high level of awareness. You will also enjoy much greater balance, flexibility and creativity.

There are several things you can do with your mind to take full advantage of its power, including:

Those who expect treatments to work, such as for a medical condition, may help to make the treatment more effective. In fact, a study was performed that showed that pain relievers for general headaches work better and faster when the person taking them believes they will work better and faster.

Know your purpose in life and focus on it to live longer. If you wake up every day knowing what you want and need to do, you help to increase your longevity.

Use a gratitude journal to improve sleep. One of the biggest causes of insomnia is focusing on the negative before bed. A gratitude journal puts you in a positive frame of mind, allowing you to sleep better.

Get sick less often, when you are optimistic since this has the potential to naturally boost your immunity. Research shows that the people who tend to get sick the least also tend to be among the most optimistic.

Imagine or visualize working out to build must. This might sound strange, but some studies have been done looking at this. One showed that a 24 percent increase in strength was achieved by those who simply worked out via visualization.

Use meditation to slow the aging process. This is no surprise since stress ages you and meditation works to alleviate stress.

Make sure to laugh loud and often to decrease the risk of heart disease. When you laugh, stress hormones are decreasing, according to multiple studies.

Research shows laughing can also decrease artery inflammation and improve your good cholesterol.

ENERGY HEALING

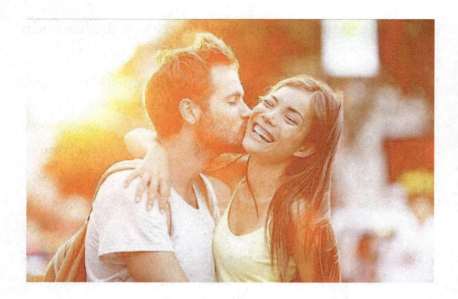

You can see that the mind can positively impact all areas of your health and life when you know how to use it. Now that you know the potential, it is time to start harnessing it. The following help to make this possible:

- Keep an open mind at all times
- Be clear about your life's passions and have passion for everything
- Avoid rigid beliefs, judgment, prejudice and anything else that can close down an open feedback loop
- Make sure that you always consider other points of view
- For conscious choices, always taking responsibility
- Never use denial for incoming data to censor it

- Look at guilt, shame and other psychological blocks, identify them and find ways to block their control over your thoughts and mind
- Make sure that you are truly emotionally free
- Spend time every day being willing to redefine your values, thoughts and your total being
- Never keep secrets
- Let the past go, learn from it and never regret it
- Never be fearful of the future, but instead embrace the possibilities

Breathing and be aware of it is an important element concerning being mindful. Find a place where you can sit comfortably that is quiet and free from distractions. Close your eyes and focus on your breathing. Listen to the gentle sound that happens when you exhale. Open your eyes and watch as your chest rises and falls with every breath. Remember the mantra, "breathe in, breathe out" and you go through the process. Try to clear your mind of everything except the focus on your breathing.

ENERGY HEALING

Conclusion

Thank you for making it through to the end of Kundalini Awakening, I hope it was informative and provided the information you needed to achieve higher spiritual awakening, peace of mind, healing, understanding, and the knowledge necessary to begin you down your magnificent path of Divine healing. No matter where you are in your journey of awakening, I hope that you achieve true happiness and peace of both mind and soul.

I also hope that Kundalini Awakening will encourage readers to reach out to others and help build a better community by applying the teachings of the Kundalini lifestyle in our daily lives. May the light you bring to others shine bright and strengthen the flame of those who burn weakest. If we follow the guidance of our Kundalini and trust our spiritual judgment, the awakening of the third eye and exploration of the Fifth Plane will become an easy achievement. Now that you have learned the magnificent power of manifestation and the positive effects it can have on our lives, I hope that you will continue to enhance your spiritual ability and continue your journey into the magnificent world of Kundalini health and awakening.

The next step is to apply everything that you have learned and start developing your psychic abilities and awakening the Kundalini. Continuing forward through ascension starts with creating the practices outlined in the book. Seek out yoga practices and meditations that will keep your creation consciousness flowing. Practice breathing exercises whenever you can. Continue to

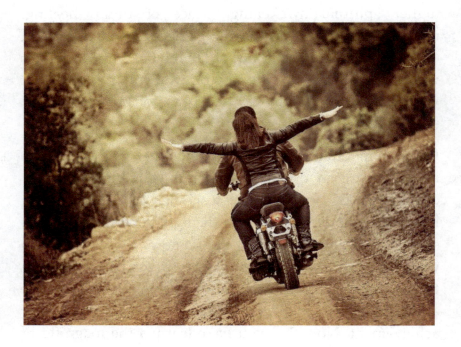

evolve and transform your alignment and chakra balancing. If you have already begun your Kundalini awakening experience, I guarantee you are not alone.

There are people everywhere exploring this journey. It is up to you to go forward on the path to finding the power of the divine within you. The journey is not always easy, but it is worth it. This is just the beginning and there is so much to uncover along the way. Now that you have gained some knowledge about the practices and effects of kundalini awakening, I hope that you are ready to commit to your journey so that you can live awakened, opened, and enlightened.

That this book can help you to improve your life.